Breaking Acne Rules

Edwin Ishoo, MD

outskirts
press

Breaking Clear
Breaking Acne Rules
All Rights Reserved.
Copyright © 2020 Edwin Ishoo, MD
v5.0

The opinions expressed in this manuscript are solely the opinions of the author and do not represent the opinions or thoughts of the publisher. The author has represented and warranted full ownership and/or legal right to publish all the materials in this book.

This book may not be reproduced, transmitted, or stored in whole or in part by any means, including graphic, electronic, or mechanical without the express written consent of the publisher except in the case of brief quotations embodied in critical articles and reviews.

Outskirts Press, Inc.
http://www.outskirtspress.com

ISBN: 978-1-9772-2355-5

Cover Photo © 2020 Edwin Ishoo, MD. All rights reserved - used with permission.

Outskirts Press and the "OP" logo are trademarks belonging to Outskirts Press, Inc.

PRINTED IN THE UNITED STATES OF AMERICA

Hannah and Noah, my inspiration

Table of Contents

Preface i
Foreword ii
1. Philosophy 1
2. Patient Consultation Highlights 11
3. Impact of Acne 18
4. Skin Structure and Function 20
5. Patient Stories 30
6. In-office procedures for acne treatment 39
7. Types of Acne 47
8. Acne Imposters 53
9. Acne Syndromes 64
10. Clearing Confusion 68
11. Frequently Asked Questions 76
12. Tips & Pearls 140
13. Glossary of Terms & Definitions 150

Preface

The concept of this book comes from international trends in treatment of inflamed cystic acne vulgaris based on evidence supporting a non-toxic, targeted, surgical approach. This book is meant to describe an alternative acne treatment approach to that of mainstream dermatology practice in the United States which relies heavily on topical and systemic medications. The book is not meant to be a comprehensive treatise on all aspects of acne, but rather an attempt to address major points of interest, controversy and deviation from contemporary, dogmatic approach to what acne is, what may cause it and how to best treat it. It is my hope that this book will lead to re-evaluation and possibly a shift in treatment paradigm for inflamed cystic acne from medical and thus chemical, systemic and chronic to surgical and thus, procedural, localized and definitive. I also hope that the philosophy and treatment approach proposed in this book will lead to further research, discussion, and refinement of our concepts with regards to both the pathogenesis and treatment of acne and, as such, should be considered more of a work in progress than the definitive work on acne.

Foreword

Why I started to treat acne and how my treatment philosophy developed.

<u>Lauren</u>, a 40-year-old, vibrant, active, professional white female consulted with me for facial rejuvenation surgery, considering surgical rhytidectomy, cheek implants and blepharoplasty. Had been struggling with acne all her adolescent and adult life with no significant period of inflammatory acne remission. Treated with multiple, prolonged courses of oral and topical antibiotics, systemic birth control and 2 courses of Isotretinoin in her 20's with persistent acne and significant dyspigmentation and collagen disruption and destruction leading to facial contour and skin texture and tone irregularities which led to premature facial aging. She had also undergone several rounds of ablative and non-ablative LASER resurfacing and dermabrasion and microneedling which left the skin dull and dry without noticeable improvement of her skin texture and worsened the severity and frequency of inflammatory eruptions following each treatment.

<u>Allison</u>, a 21-year-old white female who had been treated for acne with prolonged courses of minocycline, doxycycline and topical clindamycin and Benzoyl Peroxide along with birth control, consulted with me for skin resurfacing to smoothen the bumps on her forehead which she was told were oil gland congestion along with some scarring; however, on close examination were noted to be monophasic

flesh-colored bumps suggestive of pityrosporum folliculitis, a fungal skin infection which required stopping her current medications and intensive treatment to clear.

Xiao, an 18-year-old Chinese female who came in for rhinoplasty and chin implant but being treated with oral antibiotics and birth control pills for inflamed nodular acne on cheeks which turned out to be rosacea and responded to topical treatments with gel and phototherapy.

Carlos, a 31-year-old Hispanic man with long history of acne on face and back treated with 5 years of doxycycline and the minocycline came in for cheek and chin implant, investigated and found to test positive for SIBO, discontinued antibiotics and changed his diet and began an intensive, hand-on office treatment with profound improvement.

The cases above made clear to me the need for more intensive and targeted approach to treat the infections causing prolonged inflammatory acne eruptions and to minimize skin damage and risk for poor healing after surgery or ablative resurfacing. As a facial plastic surgeon, I realized that regardless of how skillfully a facelift, eyelid surgery, rhinoplasty or skin resurfacing is performed, the short-term skin healing can be affected by the existing inflammation due to pustular acne infection. Also, the ultimate result and patient satisfaction will depend on the health and clarity of the skin. This is why I gradually transitioned my facial plastic surgery practice to intensive, surgical treatment of inflammatory nodulocystic acne and the resulting acne scars and why I felt compelled to write this book and argue for a paradigm shift in how such acne should be treated as a surgical skin infection and as a disease and not a normal medical skin condition. Cystic acne is a dermal abscess which is best treated surgically by opening, draining and disinfecting each encapsulated pustule and not relying on polluting the body with toxic and potentially hazardous chemicals to clear the skin. The current mainstream medical treatment strategy is likely to expose the individual to a high level of risk with damage to liver and the GI tract and long-term endocrine suppression and disruption to merely achieve short-term skin clearing through immune suppression and modulation. Frequently, utilizing this type of strategy to manage or control pustular acne, fails as the disease returns once the suppressive chemicals are stopped and in all cases, these chemicals need to be stopped at some point for numerous reasons.

In this book, I hope to discuss my philosophy, which is based on international literature as well as my personal experience treating thousands of individuals who have presented with acneiform eruptions as well as my treatment strategy which aims to push the skin to clear the infection surgically and definitively through opening, draining and disinfecting the lesions and then train the skin to self-regulate and maintain clearance with a simple home care regimen since maintenance of clear requires the skin to start from clear. I will also discuss why acne is a serious disease requiring an expert and dedicated physician specializing in acne to treat it and dispel common and potentially harmful myths and misunderstandings as well as sharing helpful tips to keep skin healthy and clear after completion of the intensive treatment.

My goal is to present a treatment alternative for inflamed nodulocystic acne and for this book to be a resource for both the acne-burdened individuals and the medical providers they seek for help. My hope is that this book can be used to change the conversation in the medical community about how best to treat cystic acne without causing micro- or macro-pollution through use of toxic chemicals, hormones and antibiotics and ultimately adopt a more definitive and intensive approach to clearing a surgical infection directed at the skin, where the disease is. I hope that over time, health insurance reimbursement follows the safest and best treatment outcome instead of physicians tailoring treatments based on reimbursement.

CHAPTER 1

Philosophy

WHAT I BELIEVE causes inflammatory cystic acne and how best to treat it.

Acne is an extremely challenging disease to control and manage as a chronic disease, but may be easier to clear definitively as an acute infection. Theories as to how an acne lesion forms remain controversial as do the potential causes and even the definition of what is acne. Comedones form as a result of oil buildup within a blocked pilosebaceous pore, theorized to be due to retention hyperkeratosis, or normal shedding of the skin combined with sebum to form a sludge that blocks the neck of the pore. These lesions are also occasionally referred to as non-inflammatory acne which most likely have subclinical inflammation as opposed to lack of inflammation on cellular level. There is generally no redness, tenderness or purulent collection. These lesions do not generally cause scarring or pigmentation. Whereas, inflammatory cysts, nodules and pustules are formed due to bacterial infection of the sebaceous gland or the pilosebaceous unit and behave as an abscess triggering an inflammatory response which causes collagen disruption, dysregulation and destruction leading to scarring and discoloration of the skin. Comedones and inflamed pustules do not seem to be on a continuum or a spectrum as many have proposed as there are reports that less than 20% of inflamed cysts, nodules or pustules erupt where there was previously a whitehead or blackhead comedone. Inflamed, cystic eruptions are sometimes referred to as "macro-comedones" which I believe to be misleading. I do not believe that cysts, nodules and pustules are the same pathology or on the same continuum or spectrum as comedones (i.e. blackheads and whiteheads) which are likely caused by retention hyperkeratosis; whereas, an abscess is caused primarily by an infection of the skin, pilosebaceous complex or non-hair bearing sebaceous glands with inflammation being a secondary event due to the skin's local immune response to the foreign or parasitic organism. There is increasing data from international literature that inflamed cystic eruptions are due to different strains of *P. acnes* than the strain that comprises the normal human skin flora. It is also reported that antibiotic resistant strains of *P. acnes* are found in nearly 40% of individuals with inflamed cystic acne who have never previously been treated with antibiotics. These findings support the theory that cystic acne is first and primarily an infection and it is contagious amongst individuals and from one area to another as well as possibly from inanimate objects that come into close contact with the skin.

There are several theories as to how and why pustules form. The leading theories at this time are Squalene oxidation and consequent inflammation without the need for a bacterial infection as well as infection or colonization of skin oil glands (with or without hair follicle) by an opportunistic, virulent and contagious strain of **Cutibacterium acnes** (formerly **Propionibacterium acnes or *P. acnes***) which is a relatively slow-growing, typically aerotolerant anaerobic, Gram-positive bacterium (rod) that colonize the sebaceous gland and feed off the triglycerides in the sebum and form the normal flora of human skin and is responsible for the formation of the skin's acid mantle to defend against colonization or infection by other virulent and pathogenic organisms. Based on my personal experience and extensive review of the literature, I believe that the majority of nodulocystic and pustular eruptions referred to as inflammatory cystic acne are due to an opportunistic infection by pathogenic strains of *P. acnes*, similar to opportunistic infections by a virulent and pathogenic strain of Streptococcus causing "strep throat" or Staphylococcus causing Impetigo or MRSA. **Acne is basically an encapsulated bacterial infection of the pilosebaceous unit and the skin's oil glands.** These lesions occur with more frequency now due to growing trend of high density living and large scale migrations all around the world as well as over use and abuse of topical and systemic antibiotics in the treatment of acne. As the skin is exposed to more unfamiliar floral or pathogenic bacteria, the skin's local immune response will react to these new organisms through mounting an inflammatory response. The implication is that **inflammatory cystic acne caused by bacterial infection is contagious and if the infection is not cleared, it begins to spread and infect the adjacent oil glands and may be transmitted to other individuals with whom there is significant skin-to-skin contact.** This is supported by literature in which a specific pathogenic strain of *P. acnes* bacteria has been isolated in the majority of pustular acne lesions but not from clear and healthy skin or comedones. It is also reported that antibiotic resistant bacteria have been isolated from acne lesions in up to 40% of individuals who were not previously treated with antibiotics.

Incidence of acne is on the rise despite more OTC and prescription drugs for acne available now than ever before. In my opinion, inflammatory cystic acne is an infection which is due to more aggressive, virulent and opportunistic strain of *P. acnes* bacteria, which spreads faster and more freely in high density living in urban centers, high schools, college dormitories or packed offices similar to any other biological pathogen. This phenomenon of rapid and aggressive spread of disease in high density living is also seen with infections such as chicken pox and measles in young children, Strep Throat in high school students and infectious Mononucleosis in colleges, Multidrug Resistant Staph. Aureus (MRSA) colonization or infection in healthcare workers and institutionalized individuals, Influenza Virus infection in all individuals living and working in large, densely populated urban areas. Just as these infections are treated effectively and definitively after proper diagnosis, I believe so can the majority of nodulocystic and pustular acne lesions.

These types of infections are contagious and due to shared bacteria not heredity, diet or exercise; although, all these factors may predispose the individual to the infection or modulate the immune reaction as to the severity of presentation and should not be dismissed as unrelated or irrelevant in a comprehensive approach to achieving and maintain a clear and healthy skin. If properly diagnosed and treated intensively and targeted with appropriate procedures by an experienced physician, the disease can be cleared effectively and definitively without turning it into a chronic disease with topical and systemic chemicals which at best hope to manage or control the disease through suppression of the infection and modulation of the individual's immune response and inflammatory manifestation. ***Trying to contain or suppress acne inflammation will not clear the infection which re-triggers inflammation when the suppressant is stopped. However, clearing the infection does stop the reactive inflammation.*** Suppressants work by modulating the skin's immune response and extent of inflammation in response to the infection, not by treating the infection which is the cause of the inflammation. Any disease that is mainly managed by suppression is merely in remission and highly likely to recur and the individual will likely sustain cumulative skin, chromosomal or systemic organ injury due to prolonged exposure to the suppressive chemicals. It appears that currently, the mainstream pharmaceutical treatment of such acne is potentially more harmful to the patient's overall short and long term health than the disease itself. How many other diseases would we treat with medications that may harm the patient more than the disease itself? The therapeutic profiles of medications such as prolonged systemic antibiotics, oral birth control and Isotretinoin for treatment of acne are much smaller than their toxic profiles. One may then wonder why is this the case and I would suggest, follow the money and the insurance reimbursement which is much higher for a 5-minute visit and a prescription than 30-60-minute hands-on procedure involving training, products, instruments and state-of-the-art-devices. It is simply not cost-effective to treat 8-10 patients

PHILOSOPHY

per day rather than 50-60 as do most primary care or dermatology offices. There is a better option.

Despite some claims, there is no cure for inflamed cystic acne similar to dental cavities, as such infections cannot be prevented in the future but minimized. If the individual and the tissue of concern is starting from clear and healthy, it is much more resilient in dealing with future environmental challenges and stressors and much more likely to be maintained clear and healthy with minimal routine care as we do with brushing and flossing our teeth when they are free of disease. Cystic acne as an infection cannot be cured but can be cleared without systemic injury. Topical or systemic antibiotics cannot penetrate an abscess or an encapsulated purulent infection which can only be treated effectively and definitively through surgical opening, draining and disinfection. After all, ***if topical or systemic products or medications, both OTC and Prescription, could clear inflamed cystic acne, then no one should struggle with acne as these treatments are readily available to all***; however, the incidence of acne, especially adult onset, is on the rise despite the availability and use of these chemicals. There are no magical and mystical potions or pills that can definitively and reliably clear inflamed nodulocystic acne especially without significant systemic harm. The effective and definitive treatment involves an evidence-based process and reproducible method.

My Intensive Acne Treatment approach was developed over many years treating thousands of acne-burdened individuals and is based on the simple principle that **Inflamed cystic acne is not a medical condition but a surgical skin infection or disease.** A pustule or an inflamed nodulocystic lesion is in fact an abscess which is a surgical infection and requires intensive hands-on treatment involving precise drainage techniques and light-based technology for disinfection and custom formulated products to support the skin and facilitate recovery between treatments to allow the tissue to clear and recover completely. Opening, draining and disinfection is a well-established, long-standing standard of care for treatments of any abscess. The mere fact that these abscesses may erupt in groups on the face and are called "acne" does not change what the disease is and how it should be treated. Localized, encapsulated, purulent, superficial surgical infections require targeted surgical treatment. Just as a tooth abscess or a skin abscess is not generally treated with topical lotions, pastes, potions, pills or prayers, neither should inflamed cystic skin eruptions called acne. **Localized disease such as nodulocystic acne deserves targeted and localized treatment to avoid collateral damage to internal organs and to cause micro-pollution. No need to pollute a healthy body internally to clear cystic acne externally.** In my opinion and experience, the success of any acne treatment approach depends on proper diagnosis and a foundational principle that the majority of inflamed cystic acne is a surgical disease, which guide my treatment approach that is informed by evidence, experience and common sense. Current mainstream approach is to treat localized, encapsulated pustules on an easily accessible and superficial organ such as skin with topical medication which will not likely penetrate the thick keratin layer or by indefinite use of systemic hormones and antibiotics or potentially dangerous and toxic chemotherapeutic agents is a magical and mystical approach; otherwise known as "medical", instead of utilizing targeted, evidence-based and often definitive surgical or procedural approach which does not sentence the acne-burdened individual to toxicity and pollution with indefinite systemic or topical exposure to numerous drugs and chemicals with their own long lists of potential risks and complications. **If the disease is localized to the skin and easily accessible, then there is no need to risk damaging the liver, suppress or disrupt the endocrine system or destroy the GI flora by using systemic chemotherapy, hormones or antibiotics.**

The approach that I have used to clear the most stubborn inflamed, cystic acne involves 6-10 weekly extraction, drainage and disinfection of pustules using light source, chemical disinfectants and peels to create a momentum of skin turn over and purging of deeper cysts until the treatment breaks through and the skin breaks clear. Various and alternating Alpha- and Beta-Hydroxy chemical peels are used to stimulate skin turnover and eruption of the next layer of cysts to accelerate and facilitate extraction and clearing of the deeper infection. In-between extractions are performed in our office to help expedite clearing of infection as the cysts erupt or purge after a treatment. Also utilized in our intensive acne treatment program are a 7-10 days burst of antibiotics at the height of a purge as well as a short course of anti-androgens during the treatment to reduce cyclical exacerbation of inflammation due to androgen spikes and subsequent increase in oil production. The skin is supported throughout the course of this intensive treatment with custom formulated products that help the skin recover quickly between the treatments. Custom products are reformulated through the course of treatment to adjust to the skin's response to treatment and to avoid irritation or stagnation which could delay recovery. **The weekly pace of the treatment is meant to establish a momentum to accelerate and facilitate the skin turn over for deeper cysts to break out, for the treatment to break through and skin to break clear.**

Since maintenance treatment maintains status quo, it is much more likely that skin can be maintained clear if it starts from clear by undertaking a series of intensive treatments forcing the acne to clear first and then maintain it clear through compliance and diligence with routine skin care, just as we do with our teeth. **It is much easier to maintain clear if you are starting with clear and healthy**, especially on a clear and healthy system. The treatments are designed to force the acne to break out week after week until the treatment hits a tipping point and breaks through and the skin breaks clear. Breaking clear is the result of diligent, thoughtful and intensive effort, not just chemicals. Such a treatment requires customization, diligence and occasional if not frequent adjustments to the products. Using the same products to treat acne over time will fail since there is no adjustment to the treatment as the skin and the disease respond to the therapeutic effects of the product which will eventually lead to the skin's response to plateau and then drop off at which time the skin is only being exposed to the potential toxicity of the products since there is no longer a therapeutic benefit. Also, the pathogenic strain of bacteria infecting the oil glands usually has a higher metabolic rate than our floral strain of *P. acnes* bacteria. The opportunistic and pathogenic bacteria can adapt to topical or systemic chemicals much faster due to their higher replication rate which then allow it to better compete for resources such as fuel more effectively and displace the floral *P. acnes*, leading to change the skin pH, disrupt the acid mantel and trigger inflammation.

Similar to skin, teeth are our first line of defense against various organisms that can infect us. These barriers allow us to interact with our environment without succumbing to invasion by various organisms. Teeth are protected by enamel and skin is protected by Keratin. Once these layers are invaded or transgressed by an organism, the local tissue protects itself from the spread of that invasion by encapsulating and walling off the infection and isolating the inflammatory response. The inflammation is our skin's healthy and robust immune system's response to the infection and it can be used as a guide just as fever is for a body infection to determining the severity of the infection and response to treatment. Suppressing the inflammation just as suppressing fever may improve the symptoms but not actually treat the underlying disease. That is the reason why in my practice, we do not treat inflammatory pustules by just reducing the inflammation and instead treat the infection and use the inflammation as a guide and gauge as to success of the treatment. The surgical approach does not expose the entire body to potentially hazardous and toxic drugs just to clear a localized and superficial abscess just as your dentist does not treat a tooth abscess with oral antibiotics or magic tooth paste. The infected tooth, and only that tooth is drilled, the infection is drained and cleaned and then the tooth is restored. That is also how we approach any abscess on and in the body. Just because the pustules or abscesses are on the face, chest or back and we call them acne does not change how they should be treated.

I have long believed that we live where we live on this earth at the mercy of the bacterial flora that allow us to live there. All our

PHILOSOPHY

surfaces which interface with the outside world are lined with bacteria that protect us by processing nutrients, eliminate toxins and defend against colonization or infection by other opportunistic or parasitic organisms. When we take indefinite courses of antibiotics, we destroy this symbiotic balance with our protective flora and allow parasitic infestations and infections to take hold. There are long range consequences and morbidities to such systemic treatments not just to the individual but also to the public at large. When there is, a superficial and localize pustule that can easily be cleared without damage or trauma to the rest of the body, the preferred approach would be surgical drainage and disinfection of the abscess, not administering oral medication that is broken down by saliva in the mouth, the acid in the stomach. the bile salts, enzymes in our intestines then further degraded through our liver and kidneys, must go through 6 liters of blood, heart, lungs, brain etc. just so a very small portion of the processed medication gets to the pustule on the skin. That is not logical or best practice. If the abscess is on an internal organ such as liver, intestine or brain, then I would understand the need to use systemic drugs to control the infection. However, even in those situations, the preferred definitive treatment is to surgically drain and disinfect the abscess if possible. There is nothing impossible about extraction and disinfection of pustules on the skin. It is also the much healthier approach for the body and the skin. Topical or systemic chemicals are at best suppressive and not definitive in treating surgical infections, especially cystic acne. To treat "acne" with topical acids, antibiotics, bleaches or drying agents which must penetrate the thick Keratin or waxy layer along with oral antibiotics, hormones or chemotherapy which must go through our salivary enzymes, gastric acids, bile salts, liver, 6 liters of blood, heart, lung, brain etc. just to deliver a small fraction of the active ingredient to a few inflamed cysts of the skin is at best temporarily suppressive and most likely toxic and unhealthy to the skin and rest of the body and likely ineffective against the targeted "acne". We often go out of our way to purchase "organic" foods derived from animals that were not raised or cultivated using hormones, antibiotics or toxic chemicals; but then we take buckets of these products for our acne even when they don't work. The surgical approach does not depend on the magic of pills or potions but on tried and true methods including procedures and specialized tools. Procedural approaches such as extraction and disinfection, fulguration, cryotherapy, cortisone injection as well as directed Intense Pulsed Light, photodynamic therapy and chemical peels allow a more intensive and localized treatment of inflamed cystic eruptions than systemic or topical product treatments. Based on the significant long-term risks of the mainstream medical treatments to the individuals being treated as well as the risk to public health with overuse and abuse of oral antibiotics, it is time for a seismic, tectonic paradigm shift in treatment of cystic acne from medical to surgical for all the reasons presented above.

CHAPTER **2**

Patient Consultation Highlights

IN THE UNITED States, the population represents nearly all countries, cultures and ethnicities on Earth which do not generally share genetic background, food, neighborhoods etc. However, the 85% incidence of acne is the same across all cultures, genders, ethnic and genetic backgrounds which is most likely due to exposure to the same bacteria as we do share bacteria in our environment. Acne has been treated as a spectrum or continuum of disease starting with comedones which are blocked oil glands to inflamed, cysts, nodules and pustules which are true infections. However, this theory of a continuum of disease is not likely the case. Comedones appear to be a different condition or process and not in the continuum to development of inflammatory nodulocystic or pustular disease as reported in literature that less than 20% of time an inflamed pustule erupts at the site of prior whitehead or blackhead comedone. A pustular acne eruption is basically an encapsulated bacterial infection of the pilosebaceous unit and the skin's oil glands. It is an abscess, a surgical skin infection and a disease which makes it different from a comedone that is a medical skin condition. We encounter the world through our face which is always exposed to all the biologicals and contaminants in our environment. The more the facial skin is exposed to new bacteria, the more likely it is to encounter opportunistic and pathogenic or virulent strain of bacteria. Acne appears to be a disease of high density living and likely contagious. To that end, the bacterial infection of the oil glands in the lower face or the "U" Zone tends to be more hormonally exacerbated due to a much higher density of testosterone receptors which stimulate oil production leading to proliferation of bacteria being fed by the oil. This does not mean that "hormones" cause acne or that there is such a phenomenon as "hormonal acne". All of our skin is connected to our endocrine system and if hormones were the cause of acne eruptions, our entire skin should have eruptions and not just a localized area. Transmissibility of the infecting bacteria is supported by reports demonstrating that 40% of those with inflamed cystic eruptions who have never been treated with antibiotics, have been found to have antibiotic-resistant strain of bacteria isolated from their pustules. This can only happen through transmission from another individual who had been treated with the antibiotics. Evidence in the world-wide literature suggest that certain bacterial strains of *P. acnes* which cause inflamed, nodulocystic acne are contagious and spread through direct contact, colonization and infection. The strains of bacteria found to infect the oil glands, causing inflamed pustular lesions have higher metabolic rates than our floral, protective bacteria. The opportunistic and pathogenic bacteria can adapt to topical or systemic chemicals much faster due to their higher replication rate which then allow it to compete for resources such as fuel, more effectively and displace the floral *P. acnes*, change the skin pH and trigger inflammation. If the infection is not cleared, it begins to spread and infect the adjacent oil glands and may be transmitted to other individuals with whom there is significant skin-to-skin contact.

Acne treatments that try to contain or suppress the inflammation will not clear the infection leading to re-triggering of inflammation when the suppressant is stopped. However, office procedures aimed to disinfect and clear the pustules will stop the reactive inflammation. Topical or systemic antibiotics cannot penetrate an abscess or an encapsulated pustular infection deep in the dermis which can only be treated effectively and definitively through surgical opening, draining and disinfection. If topical or systemic products or medications, both

PATIENT CONSULTATION HIGHLIGHTS

OTC and Prescription, could clear inflamed cystic acne then no one should struggle with persistent, chronic or recurrent acne as these treatments are readily available to all and frequently used; however, the incidence of acne, especially adult onset is on the rise despite the easy availability and liberal use of these chemicals. Suppressants such as oral or topical acne products work by modulating the skin's immune response and extent of inflammation in response to the infection, not by treating the infection which is the underlying cause of the inflammation. The Goal is not to merely manage the infection, but to definitively clear it. I always begin every Intensive Acne Treatment with cleaning up the internal system by removing potentially toxic and disruptive chemicals such as hormones, antibiotics and medically unnecessary dietary supplements which can contain heavy metals including lead, arsenic or mercury. Using the same products to treat acne over time is likely to fail since there is no adjustment to the treatment as the skin and the disease respond to the product which eventually leads to the skin's response to plateau and then drop off at which time the skin is only being exposed to the potential toxicity of the products since there is no longer a therapeutic benefit as all medical products have beneficial therapeutic as well as harmful toxic profiles. Ultimately, if products or prescriptions alone can clear acne, then no one should struggle with acne. No single procedure or product is adequate to clear inflamed cystic acne. In my experience, it is a combination of comprehensive and intensive approach that has the best chance to clear such difficult disease.

Similar to a dental cavity or an apical root abscess, treatment of nodulocystic acne requires hand-on, i.e. surgical opening, draining and disinfecting of the infection for the tissue to heal from inside out. There are no magic pastes or pills in dentistry to clear cavities or abscesses and there are no such magical and mystical potions or pills that can clear inflamed nodulocystic acne. The effective and definitive treatment involves an evidence-based process and reproducible method. Effective treatment of inflamed pustular eruptions or abscesses requires intensive, hands-on techniques, technology and custom formulated products to support the skin and facilitate recovery between treatments. The basis of our treatment approach is that if the disease is localized to the skin and easily accessible, then there is no need to risk damaging the liver, suppress or disrupt the endocrine system or destroy the GI flora by using systemic chemotherapy, hormones or antibiotics. Localized disease such as nodulocystic acne deserves targeted and localized treatment to avoid collateral damage to internal organs and to cause micro pollution. I find it counterproductive to pollute internally to clear external disease. The weekly momentum of the treatments is meant to accelerate and facilitate the break outs to break through and break clear. In-between extractions help expedite clearing of infection as the cysts erupt and purge after each treatment. The use of chemical disinfectant (**chlorhexidine gluconate**) in conjunction with specific disinfecting wavelengths of phototherapy immediately after the cysts are opened and drained improves skin clearing. Also use of selective injection of deep, inflamed nodules with cortisone and Clindamycin accelerate clearing and minimize skin damage and scarring without systemic toxicity. Throughout the course of treatment, the patients are provided with custom products which are reformulated throughout the course of treatment to make adjustments to the skin's response to the treatment and to avoid irritation or stagnation which could delay recovery. Various, carefully selected chemical peels are used during our Intensive Acne Treatments to stimulate skin turn over and accelerate eruption of the next layer of cysts to facilitate extraction and clearing of the infection along with short burst of antibiotics at the height of a pustular purge or limited course of anti-androgens during the treatment to reduce cyclical exacerbation of inflammation due to androgen spikes and increase in oil production. Progress and ultimate success of our intensive acne treatment depends on sustained momentum of the treatments and proper skin support to facilitate optimal recovery between treatments. It is important to emphasize that no matter how advanced the technology or carefully formulated the products in any treatment, these do not clear the infection, the physician does through proper diagnosis and treatment planning and implementation of the plan with constant and diligent surveillance and adjustments. Once acne is cleared and clearance is sustained, residual scarring and pigmentation can be treated more confidently and without risk of exacerbating inflammation or the residual acne infection. One can not maintain a tissue clear of disease until and unless the tissue starts from clear. Phase one of our Intensive Acne Treatment is to force the skin to clear and phase two is to train the skin to self-regulate and maintain clear.

Various lifestyle modifications through restrictions and prohibitions of food, activity, make up etc. may help reduce inflammation in the short term; however, they are not likely sustainable which leads to treatment failure and patient frustration. Food, stress, hormones, life style changes may modulate your skin's inflammatory response to the infection but does not treat the underlying infection which will require surgical treatment to open, drain and disinfect the capsule. I find that a true sustained clearing and prompt self-regulation is most likely to happen in the context of a clean system, free of chemical pollutants. Many acne sufferers, begin to eliminate certain foods such as dairy and gluten from their diet out of frustration and based on unfounded claims by blogs and influencers on line, usually without improvement of their condition. Changing diet does not reverse a pustular skin infection, it can only mildly and temporarily modulate the skin's inflammatory response to the infection. I always instruct my patients that if the food does not bother or stress the GI tract then it is unlikely to cause increase in inflammation of the skin and certainly will not cause infection of the skin. The primary lining will react first and most profoundly causing pain, bloating, constipation, diarrhea etc. If one arbitrarily excludes dairy or bread from one's diet, the body will stop producing the enzymes needed to process and digest those proteins or sugars and the individual will become gluten or lactose intolerant.

Cystic acne eruptions are open wounds. A skin that is breaking out with pustules is brittle and fragile and cannot tolerate the stress and toxicity of most sunscreens as the potentially toxic chemicals can penetrate deep into the dermis and cause chronic chemical irritation and inflammation of the skin. These chemicals can also be absorbed systemically with detectable blood level of potentially toxic chemicals. There are many skin products including various moisturizers, serums, masks and extracts that contain numerous untested ingredients which are not properly investigated and may be toxic to an acne-burdened skin. It is best to exclude all unnecessary and unproven products from our skin care routine to avoid skin stress and irritation.

Many OTC and prescription topical acne products contain Benzoyl Peroxide which I do not use in my custom formulations. Benzoyl Peroxide is a bleach that causes oxidative stress of treated tissue and can cause damage to skin similar to damaging UV light and may potentially be irritating, toxic and even carcinogenic and likely accelerate aging of the treated skin. Prolonged use of Benzoyl Peroxide will lead to changes in the skin pH which will likely cause changes favorable to opportunistic and pathogenic bacteria and fungus to colonize or infect the skin. Instead, I use Tea Tree serum which is a natural broad spectrum anti-microbial that kills bacteria and fungus without skin or systemic toxicity.

Isotretinoin is a chemotherapy drug used for treatment of various cancers including skin and brain cancer such as glioblastomas. Isotretinoin (AKA Accutane) is known to cause systemic and skin immune suppression and reduction in the inflammatory response of the skin. Without treating the underlying infection with isotretinoin, there is a good likelihood that the infection and the inflammation will recur when Isotretinoin is stopped. Accutane is best indicated for severe acne such as Acne fulminans or conglobata with disseminated or metastatic presentation. Torso acne usually is more responsive to Accutane than facial acne with better long-term, sustained improvement. This chemotherapeutic drug cannot be that safe if the patient who is often an adolescent or a young adult is required to take a "pledge", sign a long consent form, be on birth control, take monthly blood tests to monitor for liver damage and urine test to check for pregnancy. No other acne treatment requires this type of monitoring for toxicity and safe guards of the medical provider liability. Accutane also requires hormonal birth control use which will cause physiological disruptions in a young body.

My approach to treatment of inflamed cystic acne represents a paradigm shift from current mainsteam pharmaceutical treatments. It is 360-degree approach with intensive hands-on treatment of surgical infection, custom formulated product use to support skin's recovery and short bursts of oral medications to assist with attenuating the contributions of internal organs to exacerbation of the inflammatory response to the acne infection as systemic factors do not cause the infection but modulate the inflammatory response to it.

CHAPTER 3

Impact of Acne

ACNE VULGARIS IS a common and complex disease of the pilosebaceous unit. The source of the word acne is controversial. It may be derived from the Greek *achne,* a word meaning efflorescence, or the Greek *acme* (Latin acme), which implies a summit or peak. Others have pointed to a hieroglyphic for the word AKU-T as the first written record referring to acne, a symbol interpreted to mean "boils," "pustules," or "a painful swelling". The clinical picture can range from mild comedonal acne to a fulminant, scarring, and systemic condition.

Approximately 95% to 100% of adolescent boys and 83% to 85% of adolescent girls aged 16 to 17 years are afflicted and of these, 83% have never sought medical treatment of their acne and 95% of whom develop acne scars. Although acne tends to resolve in many cases following adolescence, 42.5% of men and 50.9% of women continue to suffer from this disease into their twenties. At 40 years of age, 1% of men and 5% of women still have acne lesions. Acne remains the leading cause for visits to a doctor related to skin, and the average total cost per episode of care for an acne patient is estimated at around $700.

Although acne is not life threatening, it frequently causes significant stress and emotional challenges and disturbances. Acne eruptions are highly visible and therefore carry a distinctive psychosocial burden in these patients, who often display the stigma of acne or the resulting scar on their skin, especially their face, for the world to see and criticize on a daily basis. Between 30% and 50% of adolescents experience psychological difficulties associated with acne, including body image concerns, embarrassment, social impairment, anxiety, frustration, anger, depression, and poor self-esteem. Additionally, suicidal ideation and suicide attempts related to the negative psychosocial impacts of acne have also been documented. The prevalence of body dysmorphic disorder among acne patients has been measured to be as high us 1 in 5, and these patients are more likely to report dissatisfaction with their skin treatment, attempt suicide, and threaten health care providers both legally and physically.

Above establishes the need and urgency for treatment of acne, especially the inflamed cystic and pustular eruptions due to the significant potential for physical and psychological injury to the acne-burdened individuals. However, what is equally important to emphasize is the potential for even greater physical and psychological injury caused by the mainstream systemic pharmacologic and chemotherapeutic treatments, such as prolonged antibiotics, hormones and Isotretinoin, known to have potentially severe, long-term, multi-organ toxicity that may be worse than the acne itself. Inflamed cystic acne is a surgical infection localized to the sebaceous glands in the dermis and can be treated with a highly localized and targeted approach without inflicting collateral damage to numerous internal organs. The overall impact of acne on the individual and the community is exacerbated by the costly, toxic and ineffective chemotherapeutic treatments which contribute to individuals' emotional and financial stress, sense of desperation and progressive decline in general health. We hope that this book introduces a new, safer, common sense, surgical approach to treating a disease which by all accounts has miserably failed our attempts to treat it medically for the last 50 years.

CHAPTER 4

Skin Structure and Function

IN ORDER TO understand acne, it is essential to have a good understanding of skin structure and function which is the focus of this section, along with how genetic factors, bacteria, and biological and immunological activity of the skin affect, modulate and contribute to presentation of acne.

Our skin is a complex organ which allows us to interface with our environment, cushion and protects us against hostile environmental factors and helps eliminate internal waste, protect internal organs and functions while providing immunological, metabolic, endocrine, exocrine, thermoregulatory and sensory functions. A clear, healthy and normal functioning skin is critical to optimal function of the entire body. Skin enables an efficient interface of internal functions with the external environment by responding to hormones, biochemicals, and signals sent from many organs and tissues in the body.

Skin's number one function is protection. It is the first line of defense to disease and foreign invaders trying to enter the body or fluid and other vital chemicals leaving the body. The keratinocyte cells form a physical barrier by secreting a protein fiber known as keratin which gives the skin it's strength and makes it nearly impenetrable. The keratin, collagen and elastin-fibers give the skin strength and elasticity which allow the skin to resist physical and mechanical pressures and forces. Protection is also provided biologically and chemically by supporting commensal floral bacteria which regulate skin's pH and compete with other organisms and help skin metabolize toxins and digest nutrients.

Human Skin is comprised of three basic layers— the outer most portion of the skin is the epidermis which functions as a protective shield for the body and this portion contains four specialized cell, keratinocytes, melanocytes, Langerhans cells and Merkel cells. The middle section of the skin is our dermis which provides structure and support and contains blood vessels and lymphatic as well as excretory glands such as our sebaceous oil gland and the sweat gland. Finally, the lower most portion of the skin is the hypodermis, also known was the subcutaneous layer, this layer functions as insulation and padding for the body and contains not only fat cells that insulate our body but also macrophage cells that engulf bacterial cells.

Structure of Skin

Skin is the largest organ in the body. An average size person's skin weighs about 8 pounds or 15 percent of a person's body weight, and if you stretched all the skin out from the average person's body, it would take up about 18 square feet!

I. The Hypodermis, or Subcutaneous Layer of the skin, also known as the Subcutis, makes up the very bottom or deepest layer of the skin containing fat (stores fat as an energy reserve and protects muscles and bones from bumps and falls as a shock-absorber), collagen cells and a special connecting tissue (attaches the dermis to muscles and bones that lie below) and pressure sensitive nerves called lamellated corpuscles, blood and lymph vessels (controlling body temperature). The thickness of the subcutis layer varies throughout the body and from person to person.

II. The Dermis, is the most active and live layer of the skin, also known as the "true skin", is the layer of skin just above the subcutaneous layer and has two parts: a thin, upper layer known as the papillary dermis, and a thick, lower layer known as the reticular dermis. The main functions of the dermis are to regulate temperature and to supply the epidermis with nutrient- saturated blood. Much of the body's water supply is stored within the dermis. Dermis is a fibrous network of tissue that provides structure and resilience to the skin. The dermis is located beneath the epidermis and is the thickest of the three layers of the skin (1.5 to 4 mm thick), making up approximately 90 percent of the thickness of the skin. This layer contains most of the skins' specialized cells and structures, including: blood and lymph vessels, hair follicles, sweat glands, sebaceous glands, nerve endings, collagen and elastin.

The Reticular Dermis (or dermal reticulum) sits just above the subcutaneous layer, and comprises the largest part of the dermis. The reticular dermis contains the amazing network of collagen and elastin fibers, both protein structures that help the skin retain its shape, firmness, and provide elasticity, or the ability that allows skin to stretch and return to its original form. Collagen fibers are the most prevalent protein in the skin, comprising 70 percent of the skin's dry weight—the weight of the skin after water has been removed. The reticular portion also contains blood vessels, sebaceous glands, sweat glands, the root of the hair follicles, pressure receptors, as well as smooth muscle.

The hair follicle, also known as the pilosebaceous unit (also called pilosebaceous apparatus), is the structure out of which hairs grow. The follicle structure begins at the base of the reticular dermis, where it is nourished by blood vessels. The papilla is a structure at the base of the hair follicle within the dermal papilla. It intertwines with the rete ridges of the epidermis and is composed of fine and loosely arranged collagen fibers.

The Papillary Dermis is the thinner, outermost portion of the dermis, constituting approximately 10% of the 1-4 mm thick dermis. The papillary region is composed of loose areolar connective tissue. This is named for its fingerlike projections called papillae, that extend toward the epidermis and contain either terminal networks of blood capillaries or tactile Meissner's corpuscles. Blood vessels in the dermal papillae nourish all hair follicles and bring nutrients and oxygen to the lower layers of epidermal cells. Because the main function of the dermis is to support the epidermis, this greatly increases the exchange of oxygen, nutrients, and waste products between these two layers. As you age, your dermal papillae tend to flatten, decreasing the flow of oxygen and nutrients into the epidermis.

The most common structural component within the dermis is the protein collagen. It forms a mesh-like framework that gives the skin strength and flexibility. Another protein found throughout the dermis is the coil-like protein, elastin, which gives the skin its ability to return to its original shape after stretching and makes up significantly less of the skin's dry weight, about 2 percent. Both collagen and elastin proteins are produced in specialized cells called fibroblasts, located mostly in the upper edge of the dermis bordering the epidermis. Intertwined throughout the dermis are blood vessels, lymph vessels, nerves, and mast cells. Mast cells are specialized cells that play an important role in triggering the skin's inflammatory response to invading microorganisms, allergens, and physical injury. The collagen and elastin fibers weave throughout the reticular dermis, and are immersed in ground substance, a jelly-like fluid that serves as matrix filler in the dermal reticulum, filling the spaces between fibrils. The ground substance, along with fat, also helps surround and protect blood arteries and veins, lymph vessels, and nerves present in the reticular layer. Ground substance is made from polysaccharide carbohydrate chains, known as glycosaminoglycans which includes Hyaluronic Acid, a strong hydrating molecule that holds up to 1,000 times its own weight in water. Hyaluronic acid is frequently used in hydrating moisturizers for the skin; however, hyaluronic acid is too large of a molecule to penetrate the skin. It is used in skin care products not as a moisturizer but as an anti-desiccant which help retain moisture on the surface of the skin.

Dermis also contains many blood and lymph vessels as well as nerves that detect cold, heat, and pain. It also contains both major skin glands; the sebaceous glands, which secrete oil or sebum and the sudoriferous glands that secrete sweat to help regulate body temperature. There are two types of sebaceous gland, those connected to hair follicles, in pilosebaceous units, and those that exist independently.

Sebaceous glands are microscopic exocrine glands in the skin that secrete an oily or waxy matter, called sebum, to lubricate and waterproof the skin and hair of mammals. In humans, they occur in the greatest number on the face and scalp, but also on all parts of the skin except the palms of the hands and soles of the feet. Sebaceous glands are found in hair-covered areas, where they are connected to hair follicles. One or more glands may surround each hair follicle. The glands deposit sebum on the hairs, and bring it to the skin surface along the hair shaft. The structure consisting of hair, hair follicle, erector pili muscles, and sebaceous gland is an epidermal invagination known as a pilosebaceous unit. Sebaceous glands are also found in hairless areas (glabrous skin) of the eyelids, nose, penis, labia minora, the inner mucosal membrane of the cheek, and nipples. Sebum waterproofs and lubricates the skin and hair of mammals. Sebum is produced in a holocrine process, in which cells within the sebaceous gland rupture and disintegrate as they release the sebum and the cell remnants are secreted together with the sebum. The cells are constantly replaced by mitosis at the base of the duct. Sebum, secreted by the sebaceous gland in humans, is primarily composed of triglycerides, wax esters, squalene, and free fatty acids. Wax esters and squalene are unique to sebum and not produced as final products anywhere else in the body. Sapienic acid is a sebum fatty acid and Squalene oxidation process are unique to humans, and are implicated in the development of acne. Sex steroids are known to affect the rate of sebum secretion; androgens such as testosterone have been shown to stimulate secretion, and estrogens have been shown

SKIN STRUCTURE AND FUNCTION

to inhibit secretion. Sebaceous glands host and support commensal *P. acnes* bacteria which secrete acids to surface of skin that form the acid mantle. This is a thin, slightly acidic film on the surface of the skin that acts as a barrier to microbes that might invade or infect the skin. The pH of the skin is between 4.5 and 6.2, an acidity that helps neutralize the alkaline nature of many contaminants and inhibit the growth of harmful, opportunistic and virulent bacteria and fungi as well as helping to maintain the hardness of keratin proteins, keeping them tightly bound together to maintain their protective properties. When the pH of the acid mantle is disrupted (becomes alkaline)—a side effect of common soaps—the skin becomes prone to infection, dehydration, roughness, irritation, and noticeable flaking. Sebaceous lipids help maintain the integrity of the skin barrier, and supply vitamin E to the skin.

Sudoriferous glands produce sweat thereby excrete out waste products to the outside. Sweat is also the method by which we regulate the amount of heat found inside our body. So, when we basically want to take the heat and move it the outside, we do it via the process of sweating, Dermal-epidermal junction is the boundary between the dermis and epidermis, which provides a physical barrier for cells and large molecules.

   III. The Epidermis is the outermost layer of our skin, super thin on some parts of your body (your eyelids) and thicker on others (the bottoms of your feet). Tough and resilient, protection is its number one job. The protective qualities of our outer layer are vast. Our epidermis is waterproof, which is why we don't swell with liquid each time we bathe and why topical products have very limited penetration into the dermis where cystic acne forms. Nourishment that diffuses into the epidermis only reaches the very bottom layers. The cells in the upper layers of the epidermis are dead because they do not receive oxygen and nutrients. Epidermis consists of anywhere between 50 cell layers (in thin areas) to 100 cell layers (in thick areas), acts as a protective shield for the body and is continuously renewed within 6 to 30 days.

Epidermis is made up of 5 layers:

Stratum Basale, also known as stratum germinativum, is the deepest layer, separated from the dermis by the basement membrane (basal lamina) and attached to the basement membrane by hemidesmosomes. The cells found in this layer are cuboidal to columnar mitotically active stem cells that are constantly producing new skin cells, the keratinocytes which travel up to the top layer and flake off, about a month after they form. This layer also contains melanocytes which make melanin. Melanin doesn't only give us our skin color, it also absorbs some of that UV radiation which protects us from oxidative damage to our skin. Within this layer, we also have the Langerhans cells which are part of the immune system and are responsible for protecting our skin from infectious agents.

Stratum Spinosum, 8-10 cell layers, also known as the prickle cell layer contains irregular, polyhedral cells with cytoplasmic processes, sometimes called "spines", that extend outward and contact neighboring cells by desmosomes. Dendritic cells can be found in this layer.

Stratum Granulosum, 3-5 cell layers, contains diamond shaped cells with keratohyalin granules and lamellar granules. Keratohyalin granules contain keratin precursors that eventually aggregate, crosslink, and form bundles. The lamellar granules contain the glycolipids that get secreted to the surface of the cells and function as a glue, keeping the cells stuck together.

Stratum Lucidum, 2-3 cell layers, present in thicker skin found in the palms and soles, is a thin clear layer consisting of eleidin, a clear protein rich in lipids, a transformation product of keratohyalin, which gives these cells their transparent (i.e., lucid) appearance and provides a barrier to water.

Stratum Corneum, 20-30 cell layers resulting in a total layer thickness of about 10-25μm, is the uppermost layer, made up of keratin and horny scales consisting of tightly adherent dead keratinocytes, known as anucleate squamous cells, making our skin impermeable to water. This layer varies most in thickness, especially in callused skin. Within this layer, the dead keratinocytes secrete defensins which are part of our first immune defense.

Function of the Skin

It is critical to treat acne and chronic inflammatory skin conditions to maintain a clear and healthy skin in order to optimize its functions as summarized below:

1. Protection, keratin not only gives the skin it's strength, but it also protects our skin from water. Collagen and elastin-fibers give the skin strength and elasticity and this is exactly what allows the skin to resist physical, as well as mechanical pressures and forces and creates a physical barrier that does not allow bacterial cells and viral agents to penetrate into our body, protects us from dehydration and a wide variety of different types of harmful chemical agents. Excessive UV radiation can damage the skin and ultimately lead to things like cancer. This is exactly why in the epidermis of our skin, we have specialized cells known as melanocytes, which release a chemical, a pigment known as melanin. Melanin not only gives us our skin color, it also actually absorbs some of that UV radiation which protects us from damaging our skin. The skin can also repair itself when it is injured or torn by generating new cells thus affording additional protection to the body.

2. Sensation, skin contains Merkel cells which are thought to be involved in sensation and 12 feet of nerves per square inch, and nerve endings that sense light, cold, heat, pain, and pressure.

3. Insulation and thermal regulation, containing 25 percent of all the blood in the body, the skin regulates body temperature by decreasing blood flow when the environment is cold, and the skin secretes sweat to cool the body through evaporation when exposed to heat. If our temperature increases or decreases even slightly, our proteins basically lose their efficiency and cannot function properly, via the process of sweating, perspiration, as well as evaporation and radiation.

4. Excretion and secretion, sweat glands produce sweat which consists of water and waste products such as urea for detoxification as well as our ions such as sodium which are secreted and excreted onto the surface via sweat pores and then the heat that rises from the blood vessels moving that blood along the dermis is used to actually vaporize that water from our body and from the surface of our skin to cool the body and help maintain a constant core temperature.

5. Immunity, skin contains highly specialized immune cells which are able to detect, identify, and help defend against foreign invaders, irritants, and pathogenic organisms. Langerhans cells are found within the epidermis and are responsible for interacting with T-cells to trigger our general immune response and protect the body from invading organisms. On top of that, the hypodermis, the subcutaneous layer of the skin contains macrophages that can eat bacterial cells.

6. Endocrine gland, using UV radiation, the energy stored in UV radiation to actually produce something called the cholecalciferol and this is basically an inactive form of vitamin D3, travels into our liver where we basically transform cholecalciferol into a calcitriol and then calcitriol travels into our kidneys, where it is transformed into the active form of Vitamin D to regulate the amount of calcium and phosphate ions found inside our blood.

7. Ingrowth, skin must be able to expand to accommodate growth of the individual. Elastin fibers give skin it's flexibility and ability to expand as the organism grows.

CHAPTER 5

Patient Stories

THE FOLLOWING PATIENT stories convey the potential challenges and complexities involved with treating acneiform lesions and why only a physician specializing in acne treatment should engage this patient population:

1. Heather, a 26-year-old, middle-eastern female developed a persistent redness and irritation of chin after facial waxing which she began to treat with topical hydrocortisone for 10 days at which time she had developed tender and inflamed cysts on her chin and around her mouth. She consulted with her primary care physician who diagnosed her with "hormonal acne" and started her on oral birth control and topical adapalene. Over the next 3 weeks, her skin condition worsened and she continued to use the hydrocortisone cream to relieve the irritation. She then underwent a facial at a local medspa at which time she underwent attempted extractions and a chemical peel which caused worsening of skin tenderness. Upon initial evaluation in my office, the presentation was suggestive of peri-oral dermatitis. She was instructed to discontinue the cortisone cream, adapalene and the birth control as well as avoid heat or steam to her face in addition to abstaining

from use of acid peels for exfoliation or waxing of the affected area. Limited surgical extraction and disinfection of the cysts was performed and patient was started on a custom compounded gel containing Metronidazole and Clindamycin in a Lavender base. She was also instructed to apply cold compress to the affected area twice daily. Heather's face was back to normal in one week.

2. Sandra, a 35-year-old white female, HR director presents with severe inflamed nodulocystic eruptions of cheeks, jawline, chin and upper neck with moderate involvement of forehead. Reports a 20-year h/o cystic acne previously treated with several courses of topical antibiotics including clindamycin with Benzoyl Peroxide and Aczone as well as Topical retinoid, Adapalene with no significant sustained improvement. Then several courses or oral antibiotics including Doxycycline, Minocycline and Cephalexin in addition to oral birth control, Yaz for 2 years with progressive worsening. Patient was then placed on Isotretinoin and Ortho Tri-Cycline for one year with significantly reduced acne eruptions but did not completely clear her skin. Patient reports inability to tolerate any additional treatment due to severe skin and mucosal dryness, gastrointestinal and psychological disturbances at which time she turned to "medspa"s and a naturopath, became vegan and changed her job to a less stressful position; however, her eruptions returned worse than before starting Isotretinoin and she refused any further chemotherapy and became reclusive and depressed for the year before contacting my office. Given her history and her presentation with severe inflammatory noduloystic eruptions on nearly her entire face and upper neck, we began a slow process of weekly extractions, disinfections, exfoliation and moisture and anti-oxidant infusions. The

first 3 weeks, she required topical anesthetic cream for 60 minutes before we were able to touch let alone extract the pustules. As treatments progressed and skin began to clear, she was able to tolerate extractions, Isolaz, disinfection and chemical peels without topical analgesic. During the course of the treatment, she was provided with custom compounded topicals to help support the skin to recover well between treatments along with combination of cortisone and clindamycin injections of inflamed nodules and her skin was completely cleared in 10 weeks for the first time in her adult life without any systemic chemotherapy and remains clear with only an infrequent, sporadic eruption which resolves with extraction and disinfection. During the course of the treatment, she was also sent for specialized testing and diagnosed with SIBO (methane dominant) and began appropriate diet adjustments which have since improved her gastrointestinal problems developed after prolonged oral antibiotic and Isotretinoin use.

3. <u>Maura</u>, a 26-year-old white female presents to my office with persistent inflamed nodular lesions on cheeks and nose for the last 4 years. Patient had been diagnosed with Acne Vulgaris and treated with several courses of antibiotics and topical Adapalene without improvement. Began to treat with Proactive and Acne.org products and cosmetology facials and "extractions" along with dermabrasion and microneedling which caused significant worsening of the inflammation for which she presented to a local urgent care and was treated with oral Prednisone taper for the week prior to our visit. After a detailed past medical and family history and careful skin examination, it became clear that patient likely suffered from nodular Rosacea which was misdiagnosed as Acne Vulgaris and subsequently developed an infection after

the microneedling and dermabrasion. There were several pustules which required surgical drainage and disinfection along with cortisone injection of the handful near the eyes. She was started on a custom topical metronidazole and Azelaic acid in a Lavender base gel compounded by a local certified compounding pharmacy along with weekly extraction, disinfection and Isolaz IPL treatment and 20-40% mandelic chemical peel every-other-week leading to complete clearing of the skin in 8 weeks. Further investigation suggested that physical activity, certain spicy foods and red wine were reliable triggers of her Rosacea and she made appropriate adjustments to avoid the triggers and continues to use the custom compounded topical as needed for mild flare up over the last 2 years and has returned twice for Intense Pulsed Light treatment for sporadic moderate flare-up.

4. <u>Carla</u>, an 18-year-old Hispanic female presents along with her mother with numerous open cysts with moderate inflammation on her cheeks and jaw line. Reports a 3-year history of acne eruptions which were mild in the beginning. She began to treat with various OTC topicals, scrubbing several times daily and weekly facials at a local salon with progressive worsening. Patient was then seen by her primary care physician and then dermatologist and was started on oral antibiotics and then birth control and Adapalene gel for 6 months as the cysts transformed into chronic open wounds and she became more anxious and despondent and started on anxiolytics, began to wear heavy make up at all times and withdrew from normal social interactions with her peers. Upon review of PMH, patient was observed to be anxious and constantly looking in a mirror and touching her face. After a lengthy consultation, patient admitted to constantly and compulsively

"popping" and picking at her cysts occasionally causing them to bleed. Patient was diagnosed with Acne Excoriee due to constant digital trauma of the skin and secondary infection. She was started on an 8-week course of weekly office treatment with careful extraction and disinfection of cysts and open wounds using Isolaz and Hibiclense (Chlorehexidine) scrub as well as custom compounded topicals to reduce irritation and inflammation of the skin. Patient was also provided with a gel face mask which she was instructed to chill in freezer and apply to her skin twice daily in the morning after her shower and in the evening after coming home from school. She was also advised to minimize use of mirrors and to remove them from her bedroom. Her wounds healed fully at the end of 8 weeks, she began to be much more mindful and careful about picking or even touching her skin and she discontinued her anxiolytic med at 6 months.

5. <u>Florence</u>, a 21-year-old Black female presents for treatment of persistent acne on her forehead, "bumpy forehead", for the last 2 years. Comprehensive office consultation consisting of review of PMH revealed that patient had been prescribed topical clindamycin, retinoids and Benzoyl Peroxide which she continues to use. Review of pictures of her skin over the last year demonstrated a few scattered comedones at the beginning with low grade inflammation; however, current skin examination revealed numerous monophasic, uniform, flesh-colored papules and pustules which patient described as "itchy" with mild erythema due to rubbing and scratching consistent with Pityrosporum folliculitis. Patient was instructed to stop the use of her current acne topicals. She was started on our intensive treatments consisting of extraction and disinfection with Isolaz photopneumatic

treatment and Hibiclense scrub along with custom formulated topical containing clotrimazole and tea tree applied twice daily and cleaning of the skin with apple cider vinegar wipes twice daily leading to complete clearance in 4 weeks. Patient's skin remained clear with daily witch hazel wash and 2% Salicylic acid wipes with no further need for intensive treatment.

6. Lucy, 24-year-old Chinese female presents for treatment of large inflamed pustules which erupted on her chin over the last 3 months after she was treated at a medspa for mild acne with "facial" and dermabrasion with increasing inflammation, tenderness and purulent discharge. Consultation and review of PMH also revealed patient was seen by her pcp and prescribed doxycycline for "acne" which reduced the acute tenderness; however, patient then developed several smaller pustules on her chin which continued to worsen after stopping doxycycline. Upon examination, the lesions were erythematous with moderate induration and fluctuance covered with honey-colored crusting consistent with Impetigo which is a highly contagious staph infection. Cysts were cleaned, extracted and disinfected with hibiclense scrub. Patient was also started on Bactrim DS and seen in follow up with skin treatments weekly for the next 2 weeks with complete clearance.

7. Francisco, a 38-year-old Hispanic male presents for treatment of mild to moderate wide spread facial "acne". Comprehensive review of PMH and social history during the office consultation reveal that he has been experiencing the eruptions for the last 5 years since his immigration to Boston from Panama. He is an outdoor enthusiast who hikes and cross country skis year-round, has no other

illnesses and takes no medications other than 2 rounds of antibiotics and various acne topical products, including retinoids, Benzoyl Peroxide and OTC astringents and cleansers over the last 3 years as his skin condition has worsened. He also admits to frequent application of sunscreen during his outings which frequently worsen his eruptions for days after. Most recently, his dermatologist recommended Isotretinoin which he declined and now presents for second opinion. Careful skin examination revealed small 1-3mm diameter white and yellow eruptions mostly on forehead and cheeks, most with an indented central hair follicle consistent with sebaceous hyperplasia likely due to chronic sun exposure and frequent sunscreen and moisturizer use. Patient is instructed to stop using his current skin care products and discontinue frequent washing and scrubbing of his skin. He is advised to use proper sun protective clothing including hats when planning outdoor events. He was then treated with an initial extraction and disinfection of the lesions using Hibiclense followed with 3 courses of PhotoDynamic Therapy using Levulon and Blue light over the next 3 months along with use of compounded products containing tea tree serum and zinc sulfur daily with strict sun avoidance. Patient's skin cleared in 4 months and all treatments except for custom compounded product were discontinued and his skin has remained clear for the last 18 months.

8. <u>Hellen</u>, a 28-year-old white female presents with acne breakouts on her chin and jawline over the last 10 years since starting college and beyond, causing frustration and embarrassment which she feels has impaired her social and professional progress. Throughout her teenage years, her skin was always clear. She is now needing to wear makeup to cover up her acne and desperately wants to

get her old skin back. In the past, she had been treated with several courses of Doxycycline and Minocycline and used a benzoyl peroxide /clindamycin combination gel for the past year without significant improvement. More specifically, she experienced the cystic acne flare each month a few days prior to her period and the cysts would persist throughout the rest of the month to a varying degree of inflammation. Five years prior to her appointment, she began taking the oral contraceptive pill Junel FE. She reports that she experienced 50% improvement after starting the pill, though her premenstrual flares continued. She discontinued her birth control one year ago due to emotional disturbances she attributes to the pill and hopes to become pregnant over the following year and does not wish to go back on hormones. Treatment: After a complete evaluation, she was started on a weekly intensive acne treatment, involving meticulous extractions and disinfections for 8 weeks in addition to an oral medication called Spironolactone, a mineralocorticoid hormone, which acts to reduce the testosterone stimulation of oil glands by blocking the receptors on the skin. Spironolactone does have some potential side effects including increased urination and occasional irregular periods or breast tenderness. Hellen experienced no side effects while on the medication. After eight weeks, Hellen's face was completely clear with minimal sporadic premenstrual breakouts. After three months, she was no longer experiencing any premenstrual breakouts and was completely clear and she tapered off to topical spironolactone and our organic topical skin care products.

9. Malcolm, a 32-year-old white man presented with a 10-year h/o numerous, asymptomatic and inflamed, skin-colored lesions on chest which had slowly worsened.

He reports a previous history of being treated with oral isotretinoin with mild and temporary improvement. Examination revealed numerous, soft, skin-colored, cystic papules, pustules and nodules diffusely distributed on chest and side of torso. Based on presentation, Malcolm was diagnosed with Steatocytoma multiplex (SM) – a malformation of pilosebaceous unit which are mid-dermal cysts lined by eosinophils. Differential diagnosis includes: syringomas, lipomatosis, neurofibromatosis, leiomyomas, eruptive villus hair cysts, milia, epidermal inclusion cysts, trichilemmal cysts, Gardner syndrome. Sebaceous glands exist in cyst wall. Cysts contain keratin, villus hair and sebum. Malcolm had both the asymptomatic and suppurative variants of the disease. Inflamed SM may simulate Hidradenitis Suppurativa and Acne Conglobate. Typically, lesions are deep in the dermis. Malcolm underwent 8 weekly courses of intensive, hands-on treatments including needle aspiration, extraction and drainage, corticosteroids injections, cryotherapy and LASER ablation along with a 3-week course of Doxycycline 100mg and was cleared of all active lesions at the end of this course with only residual remnant scarring present.

CHAPTER 6

In-office procedures for acne treatment

AS I HAVE previously stated, inflamed cystic acne or pustules are surgical infections which are best treated with procedures directed to open, drain and disinfect the abscess. Simple physical modalities such as comedone extraction and intralesional steroid injections have been utilized in the treatment of cystic acne for many years. Recently, new procedures including light-based technologies have become available which provide a unique set of advantages for certain patient populations. These therapies provide alternative options for patients who find it difficult to adhere to traditional oral or topical acne therapies, are concerned over adverse effects of systemic therapy, or for whom traditional therapies fall short in efficacy. In a climate where antibiotic resistance is increasing and isotretinoin therapy has become heavily regulated and scrutinized and hormonal therapy is found to have negative impact on female endocrine function and fertility, such procedural treatment alternatives have become more and more desirable. This section will focus on procedural techniques we use in our intensive approach for treatment of inflamed cystic acne lesions including extraction, intralesional injections, chemical peels, lights, photodynamic therapy and Cryotherapy.

COMEDONE EXTRACTION

Physical removal of individual comedones not only has been popular among dermatologists but is also a technique commonly employed by many estheticians. Comedone extraction entails the opening of cyst with a small, sharp lancet and then the application of simple mechanical pressure using a comedone extractor to drain or express the contents of the abscess. Meticulous and diligent extraction along with disinfection lead to a reduction in the number of future inflamed lesions and an immediate improvement. However, if the procedure is not properly performed with a small sharp opening of the cyst prior to extrusion, it may cause tissue damage, making cystic lesions worse and potentially inciting inflammation by rupturing the contents of a comedone through the base of the follicle into the dermis. When performed properly with the entire cyst epithelium being disinfected, new lesions do not reform. Consequently, extraction combined with intensive disinfection, has the potential to completely eradicate inflamed cystic eruptions. Care should be taken to use minimal force, as this will minimize skin trauma and the risk of scarring.

INTRALESIONAL INJECTIONS

One of the most common procedures used to rapidly shrink inflammatory nodules is the use of intralesional corticosteroid injections. This modality is indicated for large, stubborn lesions or when a rapid response is desired. Concentrations of 1-3 mg/mL or less of triamcinolone acetonide are commonly used, and it has been demonstrated that concentrations as low as 0.63 mg/mL are just as effective as higher concentrations of 2.5 mg/ml. However, it is important to note that the quantity injected together with the concentration used is of paramount importance, rather than simply relying on a threshold concentration as a guide. I generally inject 0.1 ml of a 5mg/mL concentration with a 31-g needle directly into the lesion until the most subtle blanching is visualized. I also will frequently combine the cortisone with 0.5 ml of Clindamycin 150 mg/ml when injecting acutely inflamed, tender and enlarging lesions to deliver not only anti-inflammatory but also antibacterial treatments. Following injection, nodules have been noted to flatten in 48 to 72 hours. This procedure is not without risks and should be used judiciously in appropriate circumstances. Most common and relevant risks include atrophy, telangiectasias, and pigmentary alterations. Although studies are lacking, most obstetricians feel comfortable with the use of occasional intralesional injections during the second and third trimesters of pregnancy so long as the total dose and frequency of injections stay within reason.

CHEMICAL PEELS

Chemical peeling involves the application of an acidic chemical to induce an accelerated form of exfoliation by causing a superficial or medium depth burn. Light peeling agents result in sloughing of cells in the stratum corneum, while deeper peeling agents create necrosis and inflammation in the epidermis or even as deep as the reticular dermis. However, even very superficial peels that remove stratum corneum only, can stimulate the epidermis to turn over and push out the next layer as well as stimulate deposition of new collagen and glycosaminoglycans in the dermis which not only help purge the skin of deeper acne lesions but also improve acne-related atrophic scarring and pigmentation.

Salicylic Acid

Salicylic acid is a β-hydroxy acid safe to use in all Fitzpatrick skin types and ideally suited for acne because of its keratolytic and anti-inflammatory properties. Even concentrations as low as 0.5% to 3% of salicylic acid have been demonstrated to speed the resolution of inflammatory acne lesions and decrease the formation of comedones. Salicylic acid is lipophilic and thus penetrates the pilosebaceous unit with ease. When used in 20% to 30% concentrations as an in-office peeling agent, it is usually applied in 3-4 passes over a five-minute duration, with a fan to cool the skin as needed and then neutralized when visual or clinical end points are reached. The visual endpoint used is a pseudo-frost which becomes more apparent with more passes. Side effects include erythema, dryness, burning, and crusting, which are all transient. It is contraindicated in pregnancy and in those with an aspirin allergy. Retinoids and benzoyl peroxide should be withheld one week prior to and one week following each peel to prevent uneven or erratic penetration. Hydroquinone may be beneficial in prepping darker skin 2-3 weeks prior to peeling to minimize risk of Post-Inflammatory Hyperpigmentation.

Glycolic Acid

Glycolic acid is an α-hydroxy acid commonly used for conditions of abnormal keratinization. Reduction of comedones, papules, and pustules and overall improvement in skin texture have been demonstrated in acne patients. Improvement in post-inflammatory changes in black patients has also been observed. Furthermore, glycolic acid has been shown to increase epidermal and dermal thickness, with increased deposition of mucopolysaccharides, improved quality of elastic fibers, and increased density of collagen. Consequently, repeated peels might have a modest effect on mild acne scarring. Glycolic acid peels produce no systemic toxicity, but disadvantages include a tendency for the acid to penetrate unevenly. There is significant variability from patient to patient with regard to reactivity and efficacy. Further complicating the standardization of this peeling agent, glycolic peels come in both free acid systems and partially neutralized systems. Consequently, a 70% free acid solution contains very close to 70% of bioavailable acid, while a 70% glycolic acid formulation from a company that uses a partially neutralized system might contain approximately 50% of biologically active acid. The depth of the peel is not related to the number of coats as is the case with salicylic acid. However, like salicylic acid peels, glycolic peels can penetrate more deeply or more unevenly in a patient who is using topical retinoids or benzoyl peroxide. Glycolic peels must be neutralized, which should be done when erythema is visualized.

IN-OFFICE PROCEDURES FOR ACNE TREATMENT

Mandelic Acid

Mandelic Acid is an α-hydroxy acid commonly used for exfoliation and reduction in inflammatory erythema in sensitive skin and in Rosacea. One main benefit of mandelic acid is that it may be gentler on the skin compared to other AHAs, due to mandelic acid being one of the largest AHAs, and as a result, it penetrates the skin at a slower rate. Mandelic acid accelerates cell turnover and functions as a powerful exfoliant to remove dead skin cells. As is the case with all AHA peels, Mandelic Acid can cause skin irritation such as redness, swelling and itching which when encountered should cause the discontinuation of the peel.

Jessner Peel

The standard Jessner's Peel is made up of three peeling agents: Salicylic acid, Lactic acid and Resorcinol in a 95% ethanol solution, which are used to safely and effectively reduces melasma and pigment imperfections in darker skin. The Jessner peel is typically a medium peel, which means it removes skin cells from the top layer of your skin, the epidermis, and the upper portion of the middle layer, the dermis. However, it can also be used as a superficial peel, which has a faster healing time but needs to be performed more often to get the results of a deeper peel.

LIGHT AND LASER THERAPY

The multiple pathogenic factors involved in acne provide many potential targets for light-based therapy. Although well-designed studies including controls, blinding, and randomization are lacking, patients are drawn to light-based technologies as a "cutting-edge" alternative to standard acne therapies.

Blue Light and Red Light

Propionibacterium acnes is an obvious target for visible light therapy as it produces photoactive compounds called porphyrins that absorb wavelengths in the visible light spectrum. Specifically, coproporphyrin III is the predominant porphyrin produced by *P. acnes*, while coproporphyrin I and protoporphyrin are produced at much lower concentrations. When exposed to visible light (with a maximum absorption peak at 403 nm, blue light), these photoactive compounds create reactive oxygen species that are toxic to *P. acnes*. Although the absorption of blue light is greatest, these shorter wavelengths do not penetrate as deeply into the skin as compared with red light. Thus, absorption efficiency is inversely correlated with depth of penetration. However, toxicity to *P. acnes* might not be the only mechanism of action when it comes to visible light. Blue light has been shown to reduce keratinocyte production of inflammatory cytokines including interleukin-1α, suggesting that blue light possesses anti-inflammatory properties as well as antimicrobial ones. Studies, although not rigorously performed, have shown benefit from both blue light therapy alone, as well as blue and red light combination therapy which is how we often treat lesions after extraction using Isolaz.

Photodynamic Therapy

Although *P. acnes* is known to produce its own endogenous porphyrins in proportion to its population, the concept of introducing exogenous porphyrins that can then be activated by light to destroy target tissue is known as photodynamic therapy. Aininolevulinic acid (ALA) is known to be preferentially taken up by the pilosebaceous units and by *P. acnes* bacteria and is thought to inhibit sebum secretion by damaging sebaceous glands, sterilize sebaceous follicles by killing *P. acnes*, and reduce follicular obstruction by altering keratinocyte shedding and hyperkeratosis. We have seen clinical benefits from PDT for acne and acne inversa in the absence of significant complications.

Photopneumatic Therapy

A specialized device that combines negative pressure (suction) with the concomitant delivery of broadband pulsed light (400-1200 nm) has been developed for the treatment of acne. This photopneumatic device is the only light-based device cleared by the Food and Drug Administration (FDA) for the treatment of comedonal and inflammatory acne. The device applies a gentle vacuum to the skin surface, thereby mechanically evacuating the contents of the extracted cysts and pustules before delivering a disinfecting or anti-inflammatory pulse of intense light. This technology also stretches the skin within the treatment tip, thereby reducing the concentration of competing chromophores such as hemoglobin and melanin so that less painful fluences of the broadband light can be moved and the light can more directly target the porphyrins in *P. acnes*. Mechanical extrusion of comedone contents and thermally injured bacteria have been observed following treatment. Although a number of studies have demonstrated improvement in individuals suffering from mild to severe acne, none of these studies included a control group for comparison. The author's personal experience confirms the beneficial impact of using this technology as a part of a more comprehensive and intensive treatment for inflamed cystic acne.

Cryotherapy

Typically, vaporized liquid nitrogen or solid carbon dioxide is applied to an area of skin, freezing it. Light freezing causes peeling of the skin, moderate freezing causes blistering and hard freezing causes scabbing. This procedure is used as a treatment for acne as well as a method to remove scars and growths and excise some skin cancers. The freezing agent may be sprayed on to the skin or swabbed on, but the end result is the same. Freezing has been found to be a very effective and reliable way to treat truncal cystic acne lesions by lightly freezing the lesions to destroy the bacteria and to cause skin turn over and exfoliation of the enclosed lesions. A cryotherapy treatment may also be used to help cysts heal faster by immediately reducing inflammation and ultimately reducing any post-inflammatory acne scarring. Cryotherapy treatments for acne are usually performed once a week. Side effects of this treatment may include stinging and redness of the skin; there may also be some pain for some period after the treatment. The painful after-effects of cryotherapy may be reduced by applying a steroid to the treated area immediately after the treatment. In very rare cases, a patient with extremely sensitive skin may experience some swelling and blistering after a cryotherapy session.

CHAPTER 7

Types of Acne

What are the Different Types or causes of Acne?

THERE ARE SEVERAL different types of acne and what is referred to as acne. Knowing the type of acne, you may be suffering from is important so that your condition can be managed more effectively. Improper diagnosis and treatment may not only risk your skin's appearance but also your health. These include:

1. **Bodybuilding Acne:** Triggered by the prolonged use or rather abuse of high doses of anabolic androgenic steroids, usually used for bodybuilding purposes.

2. **Cosmetic Acne**: Triggered by the use of oil rich skin care products that clog the skin pores. It is also known as acne cosmetics or pomade acne.

3. **Steroid Acne:** Triggered by the prolonged use of prescription catabolic corticosteroids as topical skin applications, inhaled or intravenous; usually for treatment of autoimmune diseases such as asthma, psoriasis, Lupus etc.

4. **Acne Detergens:** Triggered by excessive washing of skin, which causes removal of skin oils and dryness causing

stimulation of the sebaceous glands to produce more sebum or oil which can clog the pores.

5. **Adolescent or Teenage Acne:** Triggered with onset of puberty by increase in androgen hormone production and increase in sebum as well as skin turnover leading to clogging of pores. It is frequently the source of significant stress and emotional impact on the adolescent and parents.

6. **Mechanical Acne:** Triggered by physical trauma and mechanical breakage of sebaceous glands by external forces such as rubbing of helmets or face mask, head bands or stiff collars. Also, known as Acne Mechanica.

7. **Cyclic / Hormonal Pattern Acne:** Exacerbated by release of hormones after ovulation and it is usually seen as a premenstrual flare-up of acne just before the monthly period. Acne in adult women can signal hormone problems, which should be addressed as part of successful acne management.

8. **Pregnancy Acne**: Acne is common during pregnancy. In fact, more than one out of every two pregnant women can expect to develop acne. High levels of androgen hormones especially in the first trimester can stimulate increased sebum oil production, which along with increased skin turnover and shedding dead skin cells leads to pores becoming blocked and comedone breakouts. This environment is also a fertile ground for bacteria leading to inflamed acne. Acne can vary in severity and may persist throughout pregnancy. It's hard to predict who will develop pregnancy acne, but if you have a history of acne or have acne flares at the start of your menstrual cycle, you have a higher risk. If you do not develop acne during the first trimester, it's unlikely you'll develop it at all. Managing acne when you're pregnant can be tricky.

That's because many prescription and over-the-counter treatments come with a high risk of birth defects. In general, you should avoid any medications you don't absolutely need when you're pregnant that has even a remote chance of harming your baby. Generally, the safest acne treatment involves medical extractions and light-based treatments and diligent home skin care.

9. **Occupational acne**: This is triggered by machine oils, coal tar derivatives and halogenated hydrocarbons especially by those who are exposed to them in their line of duty.

10. **Chloracne:** This is triggered by exposure to halogenated hydrocarbons such as chlorinated dioxins and dibenzofuranes through either direct contact, inhalation or ingestion of contaminated foods.

11. **Iatrogenic:** Triggered by the use of prescription medication such as phenytoin, lithium and isoniazide. It is also known as acne medicamentosa.

12. **Neonatal acne:** This is triggered by the stimulation of the newborn baby's sebaceous glands by the mother's hormones especially within 2 weeks of birth but may continue with continued hormonal stimulation with breast feeding. Also, known as Acne Neonatorum.

13. **Acne conglobata:** It is the most severe form of acne vulgaris. It is the coalescence of deep, inflamed nodulocystic acne and can cause significant pain and disfiguring scaring. It mostly effects men between the ages of 18 – 30 and can persist for many years. Acne conglobata is very difficult to treat and leaves severe scarring and permanent damage to the skin. It is characterized by extremely deep inflammatory cysts and nodules that connect under the dermis to other nodules. These large,

often interconnected, lesions are often painful. They can develop on the face, upper arms, chest, back, buttocks, and the thighs. The trigger is unknown but it has been associated with chromosomal abnormalities such as the XXY karyotype. Acne conglobate is sometimes very dangerous as it doesn't have a proper treatment so far and is sometimes resistant to the usually effective drugs used in treating acne vulgaris. Therefore, it requires aggressive treatment with multiple anti-acne medications including isotretinoin as well as emotional support.

14. **Acne fulminans:** Acne fulminans is a sudden onset of acne conglobate in young Caucasian men presenting as ulcerating acne which lead to severe scaring. This is thought to be triggered by an unknown strain of the bacteria *Propionibacterium acnes which results in an immunological reaction.* It is also known as acne maligna or acute febrile ulcerative acne. Typical symptoms of acne fulminans include the onset of fever and a general aching of joints occurs in conjunction with outbreak. This form of acne is very resistant to antibiotics; thus, it is treated more effectively with isotretinoin and oral steroids. Sometimes due to significant inflammation, acne fulminans leads to severe pain and fever. Afflicted individuals may also require hospitalization for 3 – 5 weeks to get proper treatment for this condition.

15. **Acne keloidalis nuchae:** This condition is not a "type of acne vulgaris" but it has been included in this list because its name includes the word "acne" though that is a misnomer. The specific triggers of this chronic folliculitis that develops keloid-like scars on the occipital scalp or the back of the head and neck is not known but inward growth of curved nape hairs are believed to contribute to its development.

16. **Acne Rosacea**: This condition is not a "type of acne vulgaris" but it has been included in this list because its name includes the word "acne". It is thought to be triggered by the *Demodex folliculorum mites, weather extremes, alcohol, hot and spicy foods but most commonly by emotional stress*. Rosacea is seen to be affecting millions of people all round the world, but mostly in women in their 30. It appears as a red-mark-like rash, which is normally seen on cheeks, nose, chin and sometimes forehead. Acne rosacea is often confused with chronic acne vulgaris and that is because the two types of acne share most of the same presentations. All of the lesions of acne vulgaris except blackheads are seen with acne rosacea. However, acne rosacea results in visibility of blood vessels on the skin which presents as distinctive red rash on the cheeks, chin, nose and forehead. However, the definitive presentation of acne rosacea is the nose swelling it causes. The condition of growth of excess tissue near nose due to swelling is referred as rhinophyma, which causes permanent deformity of the nose. Acne Rosacea should be treated by medical specialists with experience in managing such skin diseases.

17. **Pyoderma Faciale (Rosacea Fulminans):** This is a restricted form of severe acne rosacea. It only affects 20 – 40-year-old women. This type of acne is characterized by sizable and painful nodules, sores and pustules on the face resulting in severe scarring. It's onset is rapid and can affect females with no prior history of acne. The condition often persists for approximately a year. This form of rosacea is treated with isotretinoin and oral corticosteroids.

18. **Acne Inversa:** This condition is not a "type of acne vulgaris" but it has been included in this list because its name includes the word "acne" It is correctly known as hidradenitis suppurativa or an infected ingrown hair.

19. **Acne Aestivalis:** This condition is not a "type of acne vulgaris" but it has been included in this list because its name includes the word "acne". It is triggered by exposure to sunlight as it is a type of polymorphous light eruption. It is also known as Mallorca acne.

CHAPTER 8

Acne Imposters

SOMETIMES WHAT APPEARS to be acne is not actually acne. There are conditions and skin diseases that resemble acne, but are not and must be properly diagnosed and treated to achieve successful resolution. Many such patients have tried otc or prescription acne medications for these conditions in the past without improvement. Once a proper diagnosis is made and treatment initiated, most patients will see a great improvement in the health and appearance of their skin.

1. **Rosacea:** is an inflammatory condition that is commonly mistaken for acne. It can sometimes look very similar to acne, with reddish bumps on the cheek, though it can also present with simply redness and telangiectasia ("broken blood vessels") on the skin. Notably. Rosacea does not have blackheads or whiteheads. There is no known cause for rosacea, though it is theorized that demodex mites, which live in the hair follicles, may play some role in its development. Certain environmental triggers, such as heat, spicy foods, and alcohol, can cause rosacea to flare.

2. **Pityrosporum Folliculitis:** Commonly mistaken for acne, it often presents as tiny papules (skin-colored or reddish

bumps) and pustules (pus bumps) on the face, chest and back. They are "monomorphic" meaning that all of the bumps look the same. In the case of acne, the bumps are at many different stages at any given time. This is one of the giveaway features of Pityrosporym Folliculitis. This condition is caused by a type of yeast or fungal infection that is regularly found on the skin surface. Some people react to the yeast spores and hyphae by forming these small bumps on their skin.

3. **Malassenzia Folliculitis:** formerly known as Pityrosporum folliculitis, it is an inflammation of the hair follicles most often caused by a fungal or yeast (fungi) of the genus Malassezia which can look just like acne. It can be caused from the extended use of antibiotics, the use of steroids, oily skin, humidity, occlusive clothing, heavy moisturizers and the use of hot tubs/spas. It can remain dormant for long periods of time and then flare up with humid weather and it often "comes and goes". There are bacterial forms as well and lesions must be tested to know which it is. It presents as small, non-inflamed bumps that frequently shows up on the forehead, but can be anywhere on the face or body. It is not uncommon for folliculitis to occur with acne, but treatment must be modified to be effective. Pityrosporum folliculitis is a condition where the yeast, pityrosporum, gets down into the hair follicles and multiplies, setting up an itchy, acne-like eruption. Pityrosporum folliculitis sometimes turns out to be the reason a case of acne isn't getting better after being on antibiotics for months. It is especially common in the nape distribution (upper chest, upper back) and the pimples are pinhead sized and uniform. The rash consists of tiny itchy rounded pink pimples with an occasional tiny whitehead. The tendency to scratch spots is greatest on the forearms,

face and scalp. Most patients have oily skin. Pityrosporum folliculitis is not an infection as such; it is an overgrowth of what is normally there. The yeast overgrowth may be encouraged by external factors and/or by reduced resistance on the part of the host. The reasons why a particular patient develops pityrosporum folliculitis may be difficult to uncover and requires a skilled and experienced physician specializing in Acne care and not a cosmetologist or esthetician that may not even be aware of this diagnosis or proper handling of skin between patients and cause the mismanagement and spread of the fungus.

4. **Follicular Eczema:** This is a skin condition resulting in the absence of itchy, rough bumps around the hair follicles. These bumps can sometimes resemble acne to an untrained eye.

5. **Sebaceous Gland Hyperplasia:** This is commonly seen on the forehead and nose, in a similar distribution to acne. These bumps are caused by overgrowth of the sebaceous (oil-producing) glands on the skin. Sebaceous gland hyperplasia appears as soft, yellowish bumps that do not resolve on their own.

6. **Pseudofolliculitis Barbae:** Many men experience this condition referred to as PFB on their beard area. Affected individuals report that acne bumps form on their neck when they shave. PFB forms when coarse, curly beard hairs re-enter the skin and cause irritation to the follicle resulting in formation of inflammation around the hair follicle. Also, known as "shaving bumps" or "barber's itch", it starts when hair follicles are damaged by friction from clothing, blockage of the follicle, or shaving, waxing or plucking. Subsequently, when hairs begin to grow

back they get trapped inside the hair follicle and get infected with the bacteria Staphylococcus (staph), causing rash, itching, pimples or pustules which may crust over. PseudoFolliculitis Barbae is a disorder that occurs mainly in black men. If curly beard hairs are cut too short, they may curve back into the skin and cause inflammation. PFB can sometimes be managed with a specific shaving regimen, though often prescription medications and ultimately hair follicle removal with LASER or electrolysis may be necessary. Many men experience this condition referred to as PBF on their beard area. They tell us that acne bumps form on their neck when they shave. PBF forms when coarse, curly beard hairs reenter the skin and cause irritation to the follicle resulting in formation of inflammation around the hair follicle.

7. **Acne Keloidalis Nuchae:** AKN is a condition seen in African Men and presents as firm bumps at the posterior hairline and scalp. The bumps of AKN begin as skin-colored or reddish circular keloid scars around the hair follicles at the nape of the neck, but quickly progress to form keloid-type scars presumably due to a folliculitis-like condition (inflammation of the hair follicles) from friction, follicle blockage or shaving. Although AKN has "acne" in its name and many untrained eyes may mistake it for acne, it is actually not a form of acne at all and requires a completely different treatment approach.

8. **Perioral dermatitis:** Primarily affecting women in their 20s and thus 30s, this condition is characterized by patches of flaky, itchy or tender red spots around the lips and sometimes the nose which is often aggravated by use of traditional acne treatments containing alcohol or benzoyl peroxide. While there is some evidence pointing to

ACNE IMPOSTERS

the use of topical steroids, causes of perioral dermatitis have not been clearly identified. Certain cosmetics and heavy skin creams may also play a role, while fluorinated toothpaste and oral contraceptives are also suspected to be triggers. It is a self-limited condition which will typically resolve within a few months without pharmacological therapy. However, many patients request treatment for cosmetic reasons.

9. **Impetigo:** These pustular eruptions are caused by either Staphylococcus aureus or Streptococcus pyogenes bacterial infections of the skin which may also involve MRSA (Multi-drug Resistant Staph. Aureus) and presents as a painful boil or rash with redness, pain and honey-colored crusting that is contagious.

10. **Dermatitis (or Eczema):** presents as a rapidly growing, itchy red rash with blisters and swelling. Atopic dermatitis is often seen in childhood. Contact dermatitis is caused by contact with irritants (detergents as well as harsh chemicals) or ingredients (substance to which the actual patient is allergic, similar to rubber, preservatives or particular fragrance). Individuals with chronic dermatitis have a history of longstanding irritation of the affected areas, which are most commonly eyelids, neck and hands in adults. The skin in the affected areas is generally darker or more ecchymotic and thickened due to chronic scratching. This is thought to be hereditary, but may be influenced by environmental factors. Dermatitis may come and go for the remainder of a person's life.

11. **Enlarged pores:** Before the beginning of puberty, the pores of hair follicles are small and the skin surface appears smooth. Skin pores tend to become larger in adolescence

as sebum production increases. Aging and sun damage decrease the skin's elasticity, making pores appear larger. Individuals with larger pores may complain of small grayish blackheads on the nasal and cheek skin.

12. **Epidermal Cysts:** Unlike cystic acne, which occurs within particular confines of an afflicted follicle, an epidermal cyst is a sac-like creation in the deeper sections of the skin. The cyst sac is filled with a soft, cream-colored material that may persist or recur indefinitely. Small cysts (less than 5mm in diameter) don't usually need treatment; they can be a nuisance, but are most likely harmless. Larger cysts have a higher probability of becoming infected, which this is very painful and may lead to scarring. Epidermal growths are often permanent. Even if the material is extracted, the sac remains and additionally the cyst may return. Definitive treatment involves surgical excision of the cyst sac when possible.

13. **Favre-Racouchet Syndrome:** This is an acne-like break out common among men and women over the age of 50 caused by severe, progressive sun damage over many years. The lesions present as a close group of blackheads around the eyes and upper cheeks. However, unlike acne vulgaris, Favre comedones do not regress if left untreated and require surgical extraction or targeted treatment with topical retinoid.

14. **Keratosis Pilaris:** Acne isn't the only condition that results in red, raised bumps on the skin. If your bumps are small, rough, and look like patches of goose bumps on your arms, back, and/or thighs, chances are it's not acne but keratosis pilaris, a condition that affects up to 40 percent of the population. Common among teenagers, keratosis

pilaris is categorized by patches of tiny, red, kernel-hard papules in the backs of the arms, shoulders, buttocks and front of the thighs and legs. Occasionally it occurs on cheeks as cluster of bumps in each affected area. Unlike acne, keratosis pilaris is often painless and feels spiny and keratotic to the touch and are typically skin colored. The roughness tends to be a bit more severe during the winter months when humidity is lower, and is more prevalent in dry climes. Keratosis pilaris generally disappears by age 30, but many people struggle with this annoying, but harmless skin condition well into adulthood. Unlike acne, keratosis pilaris is an inherited disorder of the hair follicles and may be associated with atopic dermatitis. It is not contagious. It occurs when the body overproduces keratin and forms hard plugs in the hair follicles on the skin's surface. Keratosis pilaris is not dangerous, but many patients wish to improve its appearance which may be accomplished with intensive moisturizing of the affected skin.

15. **Milia:** A common skin condition that appears as tiny white bumps, often mistaken for whitehead comedones; however, these cysts are filled with keratin instead of sebum as is the case with comedones. Milia form when keratin proteins become trapped under the skin. Treatment usually involves un-roofing with sharp opening of each lesion to decompress and resolve.

16. **Millaria or heat rash:** rash that causes pink or red bumps resembling a cluster of small cystic pimples on the skin. However, they may very well be hard to touch and deep in the skin. More commonly known as heat rash, Millaria occurs when the skin becomes overheated and the sweat glands become obstructed and inflamed. The rash often

itches. Although most common in babies and young children, it can appear at any age and may last weeks or even months.

17. **Syringoma:** These are harmless sweat duct tumors which are skin colored or yellowish firm rounded bump, one to three millimeters in diameter. They are most often found in clusters on the eyelids but they may also arise elsewhere on the face, in the armpits, umbilicus, upper chest and vulva. They start to appear in adolescence and are more common in women than men. There is sometimes another affected member of the family. Syringomas are often treated by electrosurgery (diathermy) or laser.

18. **Gram-Negative Folliculitis:** Gram-negative Folliculitis is a bacterial infection that is characterized by cysts and pustules. This type of acne is a complication of extended antibiotic treatment of acne vulgaris. This type of acne is rare. Gram-Negative Folliculitis is responsive to proper oral antibiotic and intensive, surgical treatment.

19. **Staph Infections (Carbunculosis):** Staphylococcus infections on the face or the body can look much like red, swollen acne pimples or boils with pus, but Staph is much more severe than acne. One way to tell the difference is that Staph will not have symmetrical borders like a pimple or a pustule does and the pimples can open and lead to crusty skin or red, swollen skin that's hot to the touch. Occasionally the individual will complain of fever and fatigue. If Staph infection is misdiagnosed and mistreated, it can cause significant harm to the individual's general health. This condition should be treated by a physician specializing in acne and not by facials and extractions in a salon or spa. It often will not respond to typical acne

products and/or treatments and may worsen. Treatment requires prompt recognition and initiation of correct systemic antibiotics and surgical drainage of the pustules.

20. **Hidradenitis Suppurativa (HS)- Acne Inversa:** These lesions commonly occur around hair follicles and present as large, red bumps filled with pus that typically develop where skin rubs together — such as arm pits, groin, between the buttocks and under the breasts which are usually painful and may break open and drain foul-smelling pus. Hidradenitis suppurativa tends to start after puberty, persist for years and worsen over time. For some people, the disease progressively worsens and affects multiple areas of their body. Other people experience only mild symptoms. Excess weight, stress, hormonal changes, heat or excessive perspiration can worsen symptoms. Early diagnosis and treatment of hidradenitis suppurativa can help manage the symptoms and prevent new lesions from developing. HS is a long-term skin disease, which often goes undiagnosed. The earlier it is diagnosed, the better the outcome. HS can be disabling without treatment.

21. **Actinic Keratosis:** present as rough, scaly patch that develops from years of skin exposure to the sun. It's most commonly found on face, lips, ears, back of hands, forearms, scalp or neck. Also, known as solar keratosis, an actinic keratosis lesion enlarges slowly and usually causes no signs or symptoms other than a patch or small spot on the skin. These lesions take years to develop, usually first appearing in older adults. A small percentage of actinic keratosis lesions can eventually become skin cancer. Risk of actinic keratosis can be reduced by minimizing sun exposure and protecting the skin from ultraviolet (UV) rays by use of protective clothing.

22. **Skin Cancer:** Malignancy such as Melanoma, squamous cell and Basal cell cancers may be mistaken for acne by inexperienced and uneducated estheticians causing delay in diagnosis and potentially death. Most commonly, Basal cell carcinoma which is the indolent and non-metastatic may be extremely destructive locally leading to deformity and disfigurement. Basal cell carcinoma often appears as a waxy bump, though it can take other forms. Basal cell carcinoma occurs most often on areas of the skin that are exposed to direct sun, such as face and neck.

23. **Shingles, or zoster**: A common infection that occurs due to a herpes virus. Shingles is a rash that usually appears on one side of the chest and back. It can also develop on one side of the face and around the eye. The condition can be very painful and can sometimes have long-term side effects. No cure for shingles is available, but early diagnosis and treatment can lower the risk of serious complications. Shingles causes a red rash that forms a band on one side of face. It can spread from the ear to the nose and forehead. It can also spread around one eye, which can cause redness and swelling of the eye and surrounding area. The shingles rash occasionally develops in the mouth. Many people feel a tingling or burning sensation days before the first red bumps appear. The rash starts out as fluid filled cysts or blisters which may be mistaken for acne. Some people have a few clusters of blisters scattered about, and others have so many that it looks like a burn. The blisters eventually break, ooze, and crust over. After a few days, the scabs start to fall off. Shingles is highly contagious. Shingles will have to run its course, but quite a few treatment options are available including: antiviral drugs and anti-inflammatory corticosteroids, especially when the face or eyes are involved as well as over-the counter or

prescription strength pain relievers and a cool compress to sooth the rash. It is critical for shingles not to be physically handled and to be properly and promptly diagnosed to limit the potential complication to the patients and spread to others in settings such as spas and salons.

24. **Acne agminate or Lupus miliaris disseminatus faciei (LMDF)**: occurs in both sexes equally, most patients being in their 20s and 30s and usually presents as multiple small papules with central necrosis of 2 mm to 5 mm in diameter the color of normal skin or redder occur symmetrically on the face, especially on the lower eyelids, cheeks and sides of the nose, accompanied by pustules. The disorder is asymptomatic. These heal with concave scarring one to several years after onset. The scars become indistinct in about 1 year.

CHAPTER 9

Acne Syndromes

ACNE VULGARIS, ONE of the most common skin disorders, can be a manifestation and a cardinal sign of many systemic diseases or syndromes that suggests a multifactorial nature and the pathogenesis of acne. Congenital adrenal hyperplasia (CAH) and seborrhea-acne-hirsutism-androgenetic alopecia (SAHA) syndrome highlight the role of androgen steroids, while polycystic ovary (PCO) and HyperAndrogenism-Insulin Resistance-Acanthosis Nigricans (HAIR-AN) syndromes indicate insulin resistance in acne. The reciprocal action and reaction of hormones such as androgens, prolactin, insulin and IGF leads to an overlap of cutaneous manifestations such as acne, hirsutism, alopecia areata, seborrhea and Acanthosis Nigricans (AN). Apert syndrome with increased fibroblast growth factor receptor 2 (FGFR2) signaling results in follicular hyperkeratinization and sebaceous gland hypertrophy in acne. Synovitis-acne-pustulosis-hyperostosis-osteitis (SAPHO) and pyogenic arthritis-pyoderma gangrenosum-acne (PAPA) syndromes highlight the attributes of inflammation to acne formation. Advances in the understanding of the manifestation and molecular mechanisms of these syndromes will someday further help to clarify acne pathogenesis and develop novel therapeutic modalities. A serious approach to every individual's acneic eruptions requires serious commitment by physicians specializing in the treatment of acne and acneic lesions. Knowledge and

ACNE SYNDROMES

familiarity with such acne-associated syndromes as listed below may allow for earlier diagnosis of comorbidities in individuals who initially presents with acne, leading to more effective treatments.

- Nonclassical adrenal hyperplasia, with features predominantly reflecting androgen excess rather than adrenal insufficiency. The patient presents with signs and symptoms of androgen excess, which include hirsutism, acne vulgaris, alopecia areata, anovulation and infertility.

- Hyperandrogenism and insulin resistance (HAIR)-AN syndrome, an acronym for an unusual multisystem disorder in women that consists of hyperandrogenism, insulin resistance (IR) and Acanthosis Nigricans (AN). Occasionally, patients with other autoimmune diseases such as Hashimoto thyroiditis, Grave's disease and vitiligo also have HAIR-AN syndrome. In younger women, hyperandrogenism manifests as seborrhea, acne vulgaris, hirsutism, menstrual irregularities, androgenetic alopecia, clitoromegaly and changes in muscle mass, among others.

- PolyCystic Ovary Syndrome (PCOS), is a common endocrine or hormonal disorder in women of reproductive age, affecting approximately 6% of this population. It is characterized by hyperandrogenism (acne, hirsutism and patterned alopecia), menstrual irregularities and cystic ovaries. Although not fully understood, doctors believe that it's caused by insensitivity to the hormone insulin, weight gain is very common.

- SAHA syndrome, an acronym for seborrhea, acne, hirsutism and androgenetic alopecia which generally occurs in young to middle-aged women due to elevated blood levels of androgens (hyperandrogenemia) or an increased androgen-driven peripheral response of the pilosebaceous unit with normal circulating androgen levels, this syndrome may be frequently associated with Acanthosis Nigricans, when the acronym SAHA-AN may be used.

- SAPHO syndrome is chronic disorder characterized by osteo-articular and dermatological symptoms that involves the skin, bone, and joints. SAPHO is an acronym for the combination of synovitis, acne (acne conglobate /fulminans), pustulosis on the skin, often psoriatic and mainly on the palm and soles, hyperostosis, and osteitis. Treatment of SAPHO syndrome typically involves medications which reduce inflammation.

- Gardner syndrome, a variant of familial adenomatous polyposis (FAP), is an autosomal dominant disease characterized by GI polyps, multiple osteomas, and skin and soft tissue tumors. Patient with Gardner syndrome may first present with skin bumps that may be mistaken for "acne" which include epidermoid cysts, desmoid tumors, and other benign tumors. Early recognition and proper diagnosis of Gardner's Syndrome can be life-saving as polyps have a 100% risk of undergoing malignant transformation consequently.

- PAPA syndrome is an acronym for **P**yogenic **A**rthritis, **P**yoderma gangrenosum and **A**cne. It is a rare autosomal dominant hereditary autoimmune disorder characterized by its effects on skin and joints. It is also called PAPGA syndrome (**P**yogenic **A**rthritis, **P**yoderma **G**angrenosum and **A**cne). It usually begins with arthritis at a young age, with the acneic skin changes more prominent from the time of puberty.

- SIBO syndrome is an acronym for Small Intestinal Bacterial Overgrowth, a serious condition affecting the small intestine. It occurs when bacteria that normally grow in the normal flora of the large intestine migrate to the small intestine where they start growing, causing pain and diarrhea. It is thought to be caused by overuse of oral antibiotics and has greatly been implicated in the exacerbation of Acne Vulgaris and Acne

Rosacea and should be considered in the differential diagnosis and evaluated in individuals with acne and gastrointestinal distress.

- Apert syndrome or acrocephalosyndactyl, is characterized by craniosynostosis and early epiphyseal closure, resulting in various deformities of the skull, hands, and feet. Typically, a sporadic condition, most adolescents with this disorder are prone to the development of severe pustular facial and truncal acne, with extension to the upper arms and forearm.

CHAPTER 10

Clearing Confusion

1. Sun exposure will help clear up my complexion.
   DISAGREE: Many patients believe that their acne is improved when they have a suntan, so it is difficult for them to understand when we tell them the real answer that a suntan will not help your acne in the long term. While a tan may temporarily camouflage discoloration from old acne breakouts and can sometimes dry up excess oil on the skin, these effects are only temporary and the risk of direct sun exposure outweighs the benefits of a temporary suntan. For patients who think their skin gets clearer in the summer, an in-office blue light therapy is a much healthier and more effective choice.

2. Stress causes my acne to flare up.
   AGREE: Stress can worsen inflammation and worsen acne flare ups. While stress does not cause acne, increased stress can certainly make acne worse. The biological reason that stress affects acne is hormonal. Stress causes the adrenal glands to produce excess levels of cortisol and androgen which can lead to increase in inflammation and oil production. Therefore, it's not a coincidence that some acne flares up at times of significant psychological or physical

stress. While stress cannot be eliminated, acne flare ups can be if the acne is cleared.

3. Acne only affects teenagers.
   DISAGREE: Although Acne is most prevalent in teenagers, due to the perfect storm of increased socialization, stress and a surge of hormones during teen years, many adults suffer from acne well into their 30's and 40's. On the flip side, some adult patients never had acne as teenagers. It is critical to treat inflamed cystic acne when it starts to become a problem to prevent or at least minimize scarring and other physical and psychological consequences.

4. There is no need to treat teenage acne, as teenagers "grow out of their acne"
   DISAGREE: It is important for all people, including teenagers, to treat acne promptly when it develops. If left untreated, acne can become more severe and cause depressed scars. Our intensive hands-on acne treatment and custom compounded products are safe for teenagers and there is no need to wait for teenagers to "grow out of their acne".

5. It's O.K. to "squeeze" or "pop" acne lesions (pimples).
   DISAGREE: Squeezing acne lesions can lead to more inflammation and eventually scarring after the acne lesion has resolved. By popping a pimple, you can rupture it and inadvertently push the bacteria further into the skin and cause even more breakouts and inflammation. In instances where a pustule is "popped", I recommend scrubbing it with Hibiclense as soon as possible and protect it with moisturizer.

6. Acne is caused by poor hygiene.
   DISAGREE: Acne is due to a specific bacterial infection, not

dirt. Practicing good hygiene is an important part of all skin care regimen, but it does not treat the underlying cause that leads to an acne infection. Cleaning should be done gently with safe, organic astringents such as Witch Hazel and Sulfur soap and avoid scrubbing with motorized brushes which will traumatize the skin and increase inflammation and oil production.

7. Sunscreen is safe to use by patients with acne.
DISAGREE: Many acne medications and physical treatments can make the skin more sensitive to the sun. It is very important for patients with acne to avoid applying potentially toxic chemicals such as sunscreen which is likely to be absorbed into the skin especially with repeated applications due to a compromised keratin skin barrier. Safest and most reliable way to protect the skin from sun damage is to use physical barriers such as hats, umbrellas and clothing designed with high SPF-rating.

8. I should not use moisturizer if I have acne
DISAGREE: Many people believe that drying their skin makes their acne better by reducing the oil, but that is not true. When you over-dry the skin, it tries to make up for it and produces even more oil to compensate for the lack of moisture of the skin's surface, a phenomenon called "rebound oil production". Intentionally drying the skin can have the opposite effect. In fact, applying an oil-free, fragrance-free moisturizer right after washing your face while it is still moist, can help skin maintain its natural moisture and avoid stimulating the oil glands.

9. Acne does not disappear overnight.
AGREE: Acne takes months to develop and while our intensive acne treatments are very effective, they generally take around

6-8 weeks to clear the skin. Patience and diligent compliance with treatment regimen are critical in successful acne treatment. It's important to communicate openly with your doctor regarding any changes to your skin and your routine to avoid or minimize setbacks and failures.

10. Light-based acne treatments work quickly
    AGREE: Intense-Pulsed Light (IPL) in Isolaz and LED in Photodynamic Therapy for acne treatments work more quickly and are safer and more sustainable than prescription pharmaceutical treatments. LASERs have no role in acne treatment and are generally used for scar improvement after active acne is cleared.

11. Acne is treated differently in every patient
    AGREE: It is important to see a doctor specializing in treatment of acne to confirm the diagnosis of acne and determine the proper treatment plan for your particular type and severity of acne, skin type and life style. Some consideration include what ingredients will work best in the topical home care formulations, frequency and length of treatments, Isolaz or PDT, types and intensity of light used in treatment, if a short course of oral antibiotics, oral anti-androgen or metformin are indicated as complementary treatments.

12. Acne can be caused by hormones.
    DISAGREE: Hormones called androgens can cause increased sebum production in the sebaceous glands and worsen acne flare ups but they do not cause acne as it is an infection of the oil glands. Androgens are accelerants like gasoline which does not cause a fire but it will make it burn hotter and faster. This is why stress, certain foods, pregnancy and menstrual cycles, all of which can trigger a surge of hormones and can contribute to worsening of acne inflammation. However,

since the skin on the rest of the body is also stimulated by the same hormones, all the skin would be breaking out with acne if it was caused by hormones. In fact, I find that if there is evidence of hormonal stimulation of the acne, it is best to avoid hormones such as birth control pills and use anti-androgens as a complement to the intensive acne treatments with extractions and light sources.

13. It is a good idea to put toothpaste on a pimple overnight. (aspirin)
DISAGREE: This popular home remedy is not recommended. Not only can toothpaste cause irritation to the skin, it can contribute to the formation of new acne. The best spot treatment for acne is repeated cold compress using an ice cube. If the lesions do not respond to cold, a cortisone injection by a physician into the pustule, can resolve the inflammation and flatten it within 24-48 hours.

14. Your cell phone can cause acne.
AGREE: There is no actual proof but any object that can be a vector to transmit bacteria from one person to another, can potentially cause spread or transmission of a bacterial infection such as acne. Additionally, the more you talk on your phone with it pressed up against your face, the more likely you will introduce pathogenic bacteria to the skin, stress and irritate the face which can cause increased oil production and inflammation, causing flare ups. Try hands-free use of your mobile device, don't lend your phone to others and disinfect it regularly.

15. Use more Acne products for faster results.
DISAGREE: Products do not clear inflamed, pustular acne. There are millions of acne products available. If any products cleared acne, no one would be struggling with it. Using

too much of your topical acne medications such as Benzoyl Peroxide and Salicylic Acid can cause excessive irritation in the form of redness and peeling. Products are best used to support the skin to help speed up recovery during intensive acne treatments as we do with our patients.

16. It's OK to apply makeup to cover up acne.
    AGREE: It is safe to apply concealer or foundation to cover up acne on your face especially if the product contains Salicylic Acid to keep the pores open. It is also best to use a powder formulation rather than cream which would likely obstruct and stress the pores and increase inflammation or contribute to oil congestion and comedone formation. At the end of the day, be sure to remove all makeup by confirming it using a magnified mirror.

17. You should stop acne treatment and skin care once your skin is clear.
    DISAGREE: Nearly all acne sufferers should continue some form of maintenance treatment for 6-8 weeks after the completion of the intensive series to allow the skin to learn how to self-regulate and maintain the new normal and keep skin clear. Once the skin is clear, maintaining clear is much easier and can be accomplished with regular use of non-toxic, organic home care products and occasional office treatment as needed, similar to how we all manage our dental health.

18. Your diet can play a role in acne.
    AGREE: While the common thinking among many dermatologists has been that diet does not play a large role in the presence of acne, it is clear that a diet that is high in carbohydrates, glycemic index and in Omega-6 fatty acids can contribute to worsening inflammation. Low glycemic foods include fresh fruit and leafy green vegetables as well as whole

grains, lean meats, whole milk and minimally processed foods. Diet cannot cause bacterial infection in pustular acne; however, it can modulate the inflammatory response to the infection. The thinking behind these findings is that such diet triggers a hormonal response in the body that results in the production of more sebum and exaggerated inflammatory response, which leads to worsening acne flare ups.

19. You should avoid Accutane for treatment of common acne.
AGREE: Systemic Isotretinoin is not a good option for acne vulgaris or common acne. It is also not a good option for young women of child bearing age with hormonal pattern exacerbation of eruptions due to potential long-term toxic, teratogenic and mutagenic risks. Accutane is a serious chemotherapy drug designed for severe acne such as acne fulminans or conglobata or for acne that is unresponsive to intensive, hands-on treatment. Isotretinoin (Accutane) can be a godsend for some people; but realistically, it's not the silver bullet most people think that it is especially with a serious toxic profile.

20. Acne is contagious.
AGREE: Despite longstanding assertions by the majority of dermatologists, there is now evidence that specific virulent and opportunistic strains of *P. acnes* bacteria are responsible for formation of inflamed pustules. Such strains are contracted from others just as other bacterial infections such as Strep throat or Staph infections are. There is also evidence that antibiotic-resistant strains of such bacteria have been detected in acne pustules on individuals who were not previously treated with that antibiotic. Suggesting that the bacteria was contracted from another individual who was. It is also not unusual to see a higher incidence of inflamed acne in those living in high density populations versus those in sparsely populated areas. I advise my patients to take the same precautions for acne as

they would for any other bacteria which can be contracted from physical contact with the carrier or the afflicted.

21. Heat and steam are good for acne.
DISAGREE: While the occasional steamy shower feels great, it actually strips away the outermost layer of the epidermis, which can cause scaly and dry skin. Additionally, heat will increase inflammation and lead to worsening of flare ups.

22. Washing skin several times each day will prevent acne.
DISAGREE: Washing your face several times a day will not do anything to keep you from breaking out. In most cases, it will only serve to irritate and dehydrate your skin. While comedones such as whiteheads and blackheads starts deep within the pore as dead skin cells pile up faster than normal and block the pores and can be minimized with regular exfoliation, inflamed cystic acne is due to a bacterial infection of the oil glands and skin washing will not clear or prevent it as it requires intensive, surgical treatment to clear.

23. Acne is inherited.
DISAGREE: We inherit different genetic tenancies from our parents, grandparents, and other family members which may contribute to our susceptibility to acne due to a hyperandrogenic state or a compromised immune response; however, there is no "acne gene" and based on the even incident rate of acne in US population regardless of genetic or ethnic background, acne is not inherited but environmental. Since we share the same environment with our immediate family members, it is likely that we are exposed to and develop many of the same infections. A genetic cause for acne renders it hopeless. Acne is not destiny but a disease due to our environment exposures.

CHAPTER 11

Frequently Asked Questions

1. **What causes Acne Vulgaris?**

    Acne is a generic term referring to bumps or eruptions on the skin. Acne vulgaris, or common acne, often refers to comedones such as whiteheads and blackheads which are not generally inflamed or threaten skin's health, texture or tone and are thought to be caused by oil congestion due to blockage of the hair pore. Whereas, pustules (i.e. Nodules and cysts) are bacterial infection of the oil gland, which are inflamed and can cause collage disruption or destruction leading to atrophic or hypertrophic scarring and hyperpigmentation. Such lesions are likely due to completely different processes initiated by a bacterial infection or oxidation of the squalene component of sebum as opposed to retention hyperkeratosis or sebum over-production which are natural skin conditions leading to comedones. Whiteheads and Blackheads are comedones which can be managed with routine skin care and gentle exfoliation at home or by beauticians in salons; whereas, pustules and inflamed cysts are infections and therefore a disease which require the intensive attention and care of highly skilled and experienced physicians specializing in the treatment of such pathologic lesions. There may be multiple factors which lead to comedones such as genetics, diet or hormones; whereas, pustular acne is most likely caused by an infection with a virulent and opportunistic and not the normal flora strain of *P. acnes* bacteria. The skin's microbiome is formed by *P. acnes* strains which are commensal, symbiotic and protective. There is no evidence in the literature that the normal strain of *P. acnes* bacteria somehow becomes toxic to the body due to sebum congestion which then causes the skin's immune system to respond with inflammation. Our normal symbiotic floral bacteria do not suddenly become virulent and pathogenic. The *P. acne* bacteria is aerotolerant, living under very low oxygen tension deep in the pores, not on the surface of the skin. There is no reason that blockage of the pores changes the behavior of this bacteria from protective to toxic. *P. acnes* is protective of the skin by regulating the pH through secretions of propionic acid. The low pH protects the skin from fungal colonization or infection by other bacteria such as virulent strains of Staphylococcus. Comedones, as stated above, are thought to form as a result of abnormal regulation of the skin cells within the neck of the hair follicle attached to an oil gland which then causes blockage of the pore and congestion of the oil. However, there are other types of oil glands on skin located in eye lids, areola of the nipples, lips and genital labia which may form a comedone or a pustule despite a lack of association with a hair follicle which undermines this hypothesis as to development of acne. Also, despite the prevailing theory for comedone formation being related to blockage of the hair pore or the cervix of the pilosebaceous unit, the scalp which bears the thickest hair in follicular diameter and density of distribution, has far less incidence of comedonal or pustular acne.

2. **Do hormones play a part in the development of acne?**

Yes, sex-related hormones called androgens (i.e. Testosterone and DHT) can contribute to the development of comedone by increasing production of sebum, which normally protects and lubricates the skin, leading to congestion of the hair follicle pore. By contrast, estrogens reduce oil production. The increased oil production caused by a hyper-androgen state, can also worsen or exacerbate existing inflamed cystic acne by providing fuel to an aggressive, strain of *P. acnes* with high metabolic rate which competes for this food with the normal flora *P. acnes* strain with a much lower metabolic rate, effectively displacing it. However, androgen hormone spikes do not cause inflamed cystic pustules. Testosterone's effect on inflamed cystic acne is similar to gasoline's effect on fire. Gasoline is an accelerant not an incendiary in that it worsens fire but does not cause it. Testosterone spike often worsens the inflammatory response to the infection caused by a virulent strain of *P. acnes*, but it does not cause the infection. In addition to stimulating oil production, hormonal fluctuations cause modulation in the immune response and therefore effect the extent of the inflammation; but do not cause a bacterial infection. If hormones were the cause of pustular eruptions, then our entire skin would be involved and not just our face or a small segment of the skin. This is why I do not recommend treating hormonal exacerbation of cystic acne with more hormones such as progesterone in systemic birth control medications which the body can easily turn into more testosterone instead of short-term use of anti-androgens such as Spironolactone for women or Finasteride for men as a complement to the procedural or surgical treatment of the underlying infection to decrease skin sebum levels and not just artificially modulate the skin's inflammatory response to the infection.

3. Does acne run in families (is it genetic)?

A gene causing acne has never been found. In fact, there are published evidence that individuals who migrated from certain Islands without any history of acne, develop acne at the same rate of multigenerational, life-long residents of the United States or Europe after only one generation. This evidence undermines any suggestion that cystic, inflammatory acne is hereditary. However, certain inherited conditions or skin types such as oily skin may predispose the individual to more frequent comedone, whitehead and blackhead, formation. Unlike inflamed pustular eruptions which are a skin disease cause by an infection, comedones developed due to excess oil production and derangement in skin cell shedding are merely a normal skin condition which can be managed with regular cleansing and exfoliation and regulation of oil production with topical Sulphur or oral antiandrogen medications. There is no evidence which prove that inflamed cystic acne has genetic predilection. After all, inflamed cystic acne is a treatable infection, not a family curse. If cystic acne was genetic, there would be no hope. In my opinion, inflammatory cystic acne is as genetic as Strep throat or Mononucleosis infections. It is merely a matter of exposure to the wrong strain of the organism at the wrong time when our natural immunity is compromised.

I personally have not found that individuals with a family history of severe acne are more likely to develop severe acne than those with no known family history. Besides, it would be difficult to separate genetics from environmental factors amongst genetically related individuals who live under the same roof and are exposed to the same environment and the same bacteria. Accepting the genetic theory is fatalistic without much hope, as genetics is not about the past but a predictor of the future. The reality of my experience has been that the infectious, bacterial theory allows one to be more existential and believe that acne-burdened individuals do not have to accept a predetermined fate and can treat, not just suppress or manage their disease. Based on this knowledge and procedures developed over many years of treating difficult inflammatory nodulocystic acne, the future for those burdened by such acne is hopeful, not fateful or fearful of not only the devastation resulting from the acne but also the injury caused by the conventional, mainstream topical and systemic treatments.

4. **At what age do people usually first develop acne?**
It was long thought that acne is a disease of teens due to

puberty starting as early as 11; however, recent data demonstrate that acne is common in children ages 7 to 12. This is likely due to earlier socialization of young children in high density urban schools, sports, camps etc. and not as hypothesized by some to be due to earlier onset of adrenarche (when the adrenal glands awaken) and menarche (first period). It is also recently reported that adult onset acne well into the 30's is on a sharp rise. This may also be attributed to an increase in high density, diasporic, multinational living by an increasing number of people leading to exposure to more opportunistic, virulent and drug resistant strains of *P. acnes* bacteria.

5. How common is acne?

It is said that 100% of people will experience an acne breakout of at least a few pimples at some point in their life. Acne is the most common skin disease in the United States and likely in the world. More than 50 million Americans suffer from acne annually, of those, nearly 85% of people between 12-24 years of age develop acne to some degree. 15% have some form of acne bad enough that it results in scarring on the skin. Approximately 95% to 100% of adolescent boys and 83% to 85% of adolescent girls aged 16 to 17 years in the United States are afflicted. Acne breakouts peak at 14-17 years of age in women and at 16-19 in men. Although acne has long been thought to resolve following adolescence, 42.5% of men and 50.9% of women continue to suffer from this disease into their twenties. Acne can occur at any stage of life and may continue into one's 30s and 40s. The incidence of acne occurring in adults is increasing as 14% of women battle acne well into their 40s. The average age of people with acne has increased over the last decade from 20.5 years to 26.5 years old.

6. Are there different types of acne?

There are many different types of acne based on their cause and presentation. Previously and to a large extent even presently,

FREQUENTLY ASKED QUESTIONS

many dermatologist considered the main two categories of acne as "inflammatory" and "non-inflammatory". Non-inflammatory acne lesions, which I refer to as "comedones" are the whitehead or closed and blackhead or open and oxidized lesions. Inflammatory acne is what I refer to as "pustules, nodules and cysts" which more commonly lead to scarring and pigmentation. However, more recently, reports suggest that all lesions have some inflammation with comedones being subclinical or asymptomatic and pustules and nodulocystic eruptions being overt or severe. Inflammation appears to be an early process in the development of acne which may be the trigger for the retention hyperkeratosis or follicle pore blockage leading to sebum congestion. There is also evidence of oxidation of squalene component of the sebum which triggers the inflammation without the presence of bacteria. The most transformational information in the recent scientific literature suggests that the cause for the nodulocystic or pustular eruptions is infection of the oil glands with an opportunistic and virulent strain of *P. acnes* bacteria which is different than the normally indolent and protective *P. acnes* flora. This information suggests transmissibility from one individual to another or potentially involving a middle vector such as pets or in animate objects that come into close contact with the affected skin. Subtypes of acne are also based on association with various exposures. Taking a detailed history and close examination of the acne and its distribution by a skilled physician specializing in treatment of acne is critical in identifying the closest association to aid in implementing the proper treatment plan and to minimize or eliminate the associated trigger. A more detailed, non-comprehensive list of the most common subtypes of acne is provided in the chapter pertaining to types of acne.

7. **Is acne contagious?**

This is extremely controversial with mainstream dermatologists insisting that it is not; however, recent evidence suggests that the inflamed cystic acne is caused by an opportunistic, virulent strain of *P. acnes* which may be transmitted between individuals. Also reported is the high incidence of antibiotic resistant strain of *P. acnes* in the pustules of individuals never previously treated with the antibiotics. These findings suggest the high likelihood that the strain of bacteria that causes inflammatory, cystic acne is transmissible and can be caught from someone else. It is also likely that there may be an intermediary vector such as a pet or an inanimate object which facilitates the transmission. As we live in increasingly dense and internationally diverse communities, our skin comes into contact with unfamiliar strains of bacteria which have not developed a symbiotic relationship with our skin and to which our skin reacts as a foreign invader; thus, causing localized inflammation. This is similar to traveling to remote corners of the world and ingesting unfamiliar bacteria to which our intestinal lining will have a dramatic and violent inflammatory reaction known as travelers' diarrhea which may be fatal in some instances. After all, as I have always believed, we live where we live on this Earth at the mercy of the bacteria and other microorganisms that allow us to live there. When we make drastic geographic population moves, the linings of our body become reactive to the new organisms which may be normal flora for the indigenous population, but highly reactive and inflammatory to others. In addition, ever increasing strains of antibiotic resistant bacteria developed due to decades of misuse and abuse of antibiotics, especially for the treatment of acne, contribute to the risk of infection with pathogenic bacteria. This is why I advocate for localized, surgical or procedural treatment of inflammatory cystic acne as a more effective and definitive treatment of abscess-like eruptions and less toxic and negatively consequential pharmaceutical approach effecting not only the long-term health and quality of life of the patient but also endangering the public's health at large.

FREQUENTLY ASKED QUESTIONS

8. **If we all have *P. acnes*, why do some break out while others don't?**

    Based on my review of literature, I believe it all has to do with what strain of *P. acnes* bacteria has colonized or infected the oil glands. A recent study in the *Journal of Investigative Dermatology* broke historic ground with the study of *P. acnes*. They sampled the *P. acnes* of 100 people and found that those with certain strands were either more likely to suffer with acne or more likely to not have acne at all. It boils down to the fact that we all have *P. acnes* to protect our skin, but what strand or strain we have will be the determining factor in how severely or if acne affects our skin. This is why I believe that the future of treatment for infections such as acne is not with antibiotics but with topical probiotic treatments to replace protective bacteria such as the use of facial masks containing Propiobacterium strain found in the culture of Swiss cheese. Oral supplements with probiotics are not likely to be effective as they contain Lactobacillus which is not a skin flora bacteria.

9. **Why do I keep breaking out in the same areas?**

    Since cystic acne is truly an infection of the oil glands which then turns into a pustule or abscess, it does not clear unless and until it is opened, drained and disinfected; otherwise, it will continue to recur in the same location. Surgical disinfection allows the cysts to heal from inside. Normally, an abscess that is not completely cleaned and disinfected will continue to reform and recur in the same location. A pustule, similar to an abscess, is a surgical disease which is localized and requires a surgical treatment to fully clear as no systemic or topical treatments clear such an infection.

10. **Do teenagers outgrow their acne?**

    Although the severity of the inflammatory acne along with extent of hormonally stimulated sebum production, may decrease once past the teen years, acne eruptions frequently continue well into adulthood with some experiencing worsening or new onset acne well into 20's and 30's as they go off to college, to military or start a new job in a different part of the country or the world. It is important to treat pustular acne promptly and intensively whenever it presents. Waiting to outgrow acne can lead to permanent scars and years of active inflammation. Just as chronic dental inflammation is known to have a negative long-term effect on general health, I believe so does the persistent and severe inflammation of our largest organ by surface area, the skin.

11. I'm a parent, how can I talk to my teen about seeking treatment for acne?

It's most likely that your teen feels self-conscious about their skin if they're suffering from acne. Start by asking your child how his or her skincare has been going and if they are now looking for any help with it. A recent study showed that most teens do not seek medical help for their acne. The best way to get your teen the help they need is by making them an appointment with an experienced and compassionate doctor specializing in the treatment of acne. Your teen needs to be heard and reassured along with being provided with an intensive structure to help them clear their acne with minimal reliance on their compliance to start. As they begin to see progress and improve their outlook regarding their skin, more home care responsibilities will be placed on their shoulders and compliance will be monitored closely and reinforced by the doctor's team instead of the parent to dissociate acne from parental criticism and condemnation. The parent should address all their questions and concerns to the treating physician to shield teen from added stress at home and to preserve a healthy and supportive parent-child relationship. The acne physician (Acneologist) will only briefly be in your teen's life if successful; however, a parent's role is life-long. It is important to not make the teen feel that he or she has done something wrong to deserve the acne or that it is a family curse with no chance for effective treatment. Skin is just another organ that can suffer from disease and having an experienced medical professional take over the treatment of the disease is critical in the preservation of not only the teen's skin health but also his or her mental health. The right treatment plan can only be devised and implemented by a physician after spending time with the teen and learning more about their everyday life, inspirations and aspirations. The solution may be simple, but it is rarely easy.

12 How common is adult acne?

According to recent reports, adult acne is on the rise. Although acne breakouts peak at 14-17 years of age in women and at 16-19 in men, subsiding in many cases following adolescence, 42.5% of men and 50.9% of women continue to suffer from this disease into their twenties as well as up to 25 percent of women ages of 30-49. The average age of people with acne has increased over the last decade from 20.5 years to 26.5 years old.

Many have blamed hormonal changes as we age and the role androgens play in sebum production and how quickly the skin sheds its cells for the increase in the incidence of adult acne which in my opinion is unsupported by evidence. It remains my opinion based on my experience and literature review that the subtype of inflammatory, cystic acne which persists in adulthood despite the extensive use of over-the-counter and prescription topicals and systemic chemicals is due to infection by a *P. acnes* strain of bacteria which is foreign and or pathogenic to our skin's immune system leading to inflammatory acne flare ups. Rosacea, especially in adult women is another common skin disease that is frequently mistaken for inflammatory cystic acne and improperly treated leading to persistence or worsening of the condition.

13. Is there a difference between adult acne and teenage acne?

The same causative agents that lead to acne formation form

both adult and teenage acne but perhaps to different extent. Overall skin condition, the individual's health and comorbidities, activities, treatment availability and exposure to the elements may be the variables that must be considered when deciding on a treatment plan for an adult versus a teen.

14. What else may be causing me to breakout?
Not all skin bumps are acne especially when they do not respond even temporarily to any of the conventional over-the-counter or prescriptive medical treatments. There are many acne imposters which are often misdiagnosed and mismanaged by inexperienced providers, especially non-physicians and physicians who do not specialize in treating acne. Review the chapter on acne imposters for a non-exhaustive list such lesions.

15. What is Rosacea?
About 16 million Americans have Rosacea, yet very few seek the proper treatment for it. In fact, many people mistake Rosacea for acne. Like acne, rosacea is an inflammatory condition. Rosacea may present itself in many ways, the most common being acne-like bumps on the face and erythema (redness) with telangiectasia (blood vessels) over the cheeks and nose. The exact cause of Rosacea is unknown and there is no cure. Rosacea may be worsened by certain triggers, which can differ in every patient. Vasodilation, which is a flushing on the face, is exaggerated in patients with Rosacea upon exposure to heat. Traditional acne treatments such as topical Retinoids, Benzoyl Peroxide, Salicylic Acid, oral antibiotics etc. not only do not improve this condition but may significantly exacerbate it. This is why the skin condition must be first properly diagnosed by an acneologist, a medical doctor specializing in the treatment of acne and acne-like conditions, in order for the right treatment to be implemented to improve the condition and not risk worsening with improper treatments based on incorrect assumptions of the presenting

disease. In my practice, we utilize a specially compounded gel containing metronidazole and Azelaic acid in combination with series of light-based treatments using the red-light spectrum IPL and localized extractions of pustules as needed.

16. What is the difference between acne and rosacea?

Acne and rosacea are different conditions, with different causes, though they can appear very similar. Rosacea is thought to be a vasculitis, or inflammation of blood vessels; whereas, cystic acne is thought to be a bacterial infection of the oil glands on the skin. Rosacea bumps can mimic acne, often making it very difficult to distinguish the two conditions from each other. However, patients with rosacea do not develop comedones (blackheads and whiteheads), and acne patients do not experience flushing with known triggers. These are two key signs to differentiate the two on examination. Also, rosacea is more common on the central face – cheeks, nose and chin.

17. What is the mental health toll on acne sufferers?

It is very common for acne sufferers to feel depressed. In a variety of studies, anywhere from 13-38% of acne patients – or as high as half of adolescent acne patients – report depression or meet criteria for other psychological disorders. Low self-esteem, anxiety, social stigmatization or isolation and feelings of helplessness and hopelessness – all symptoms of depression – can be side effects that accompany persistent inflamed cystic acne. There is an increased correlation between depression and acne, but correlation does not indicate causation (association). A complicating factor is that the time that is most common for acne to strike, late adolescence and early adulthood, is also a very common time for psychological symptoms to emerge. If you are experiencing feelings of depression, consult with your doctor immediately. One of the most important factors in properly managing stress and depression is to develop an intensive treatment plan which produces visible improvements that promotes optimism, control and empowerment.

18. What can I do to prevent myself from picking at my acne?

If you have a difficulty controlling yourself from picking at your acne, you may be suffering from a skin-picking disorder called neurotic excoriation. These are called body-focused repetitive-behaviors (BFRBs); repetitive self-grooming behaviors in which pulling, picking, biting or scraping of the hair, skin and nails result in damage to the body. These presentations can be similar in certain ways to obsessive-compulsive disorder and often include elements of perfectionism which is now magnified in the age of social media, selfies and filters creating the idealized illusion of perfect skin towards which many attempt to strive with futility. Those with BFRBs often experience a physical or emotional urge to pull or pick and feeling of tension or boredom commonly triggers the behavior, resulting in fleeting pleasure, gratification or relief while engaging in the pulling/picking that quickly can turn to self-directed anger or guilt afterward. With BFRBs often comes shame, secrecy, isolation, and interference with intimate relationships, avoidance of activities one would otherwise pursue as well as possible interference with work or study. We find that one of the best ways to relieve the inflammation and desensitize the skin and reduce the irritation is by applying cold compress, such as an ice cube, to the irritated skin. This may be repeated as needed. Another topical treatment that may reduce the urge to pick is Calamine which will calm the skin and reduce itching or irritation. Patients in my practice are encouraged to contact our office to come in for extraction or skin hydration treatments to break the cycle of excoriation, stress and anxiety. If self-help is not enough and you believe you are suffering from a skin-picking disorder or other BFRB, we suggest counseling with a mental health professional. The website www.trich.org is a great resource to learn more and to help find qualified mental health professional to help you stop picking.

FREQUENTLY ASKED QUESTIONS

19. How is acne different in patients with skin of color?

Acne in darker skin is very similar to acne in patients with lighter skin types. Acne breakouts occur from the same factors, regardless of your skin color or type. However, other conditions which occur more frequently in darker skin and present as skin bumps especially on the face may be mistaken for acne. Some of these conditions include Pseudofolliculitis Barbae, Millia and sebaceous hyperplasia, which if not treated correctly will lead to prolonged skin inflammation, hyper- or hypo-pigmentation and scarring. Although cystic acne may form the same way in all individual, treating acne can present some unique challenges in patients with darker skin. Patients with darker skin color are prone to rare loss of pigmentation which may be permanent or more commonly develop residual dark marks for weeks to months after acne breakouts. These left-over marks are called "Post-Inflammatory Hyperpigmentation" (PIH), which can be very difficult to treat and frustrating for the patient.

20. Can using hair or skin oils cause acne?

Certain oils such as coconut oil may cause comedonal acne by clogging up the pores leading to congestion of the oil glands. Interestingly, using hair oils on the scalp may cause comedones along the hairline on the forehead and back of neck but rarely the scalp or anywhere else on the face. Since pustules and inflamed nodulocystic eruptions are caused by bacterial infection, use of such products is not causative but, may prolong recovery.

21. How common is new onset acne when you are pregnant?

Worsening of dormant or low grade acne is very common skin complaint during pregnancy due to hormonal fluctuations. True pustular eruptions are uncommon in women who lack a history of acne prior to becoming pregnant. The first trimester is the most common time for such breakouts. In my experience, the incidence, extent and severity of the acne eruption are higher if the

BREAKING CLEAR

woman becomes pregnant soon after discontinuing prolonged use of systemic hormonal birth control which was suppressing hormonal stimulation of existing acne. This is one of the reasons why we do not treat acne in female patients with oral birth control and if they are on hormones, I encourage them to periodically come off and help the body normalize and self-regulate to help identify and treat hormonal suppression of acne before planned pregnancy.

22. If you get new onset acne when you are pregnant, should you wait until after giving birth to have it treated?

Given that we treat acne using localized, targeted procedures such as extractions and light-based energy sources instead of traditional medical products and prescriptions, there is no reason for the pregnant woman to live with the persistent inflammation, discomfort and potential scarring. The mother's health always takes precedent especially if the untreated disease may cause the mother injury and the treatment has no or very low likelihood of risk to the fetus. Waiting to treat acne until after giving birth may take longer than expected as the period after giving birth is often referred to as the "fourth trimester" because of the changes still taking place in the mother's body. After giving birth, the hormone levels in the mother's body can be unpredictable for up to a year, so you can still expect flares of low grade or dormant acne during this time

23. What products are best to clear my teen's acne?

Home care regimen is only effective in keeping skin clear once the skin has been cleared of active inflamed cystic eruptions using intensive, hands-on office treatments. There are hundreds if not thousands of over-the-counter and prescription products on the market. If any of these products cleared inflamed cystic acne, then no one should be struggling with acne, as these products are readily available to everyone. Products are best for skin support and recovery to maintain clear not to achieve clear. It is easier to maintain clear when you start from clear. Similarly, no tooth paste is available to treat tooth infection or cavity as it requires intensive, localized surgical treatment to restore tissue health before regular brushing can maintain clear and healthy tissue.

24. How does Salicylic acid work?

Salicylic acid is a "Keratolytic agent", meaning it is a peeling agent that helps breakdown the waxy keratin that forms a protective barrier on the top layer of the skin. Salicylic acid also helps shed cells inside the hair follicles, which in turn prevent the pores from clogging and keeps them free of debris. Salicylic acid can help reduce whiteheads and blackheads but not inflamed pustules. Salicylic acid concentrations approved for use in over the counter treatments for acne fall between 0.5 percent to 2.0 percent, far below what we are able to use in the office under careful and controlled conditions. The negative side of salicylic acid is that it can cause stinging and skin irritations, such as cracking, burns and redness and may cause additional skin injury if used to treat other lesions misdiagnosed as comedones.

25. How does Benzoyl Peroxide (BPO) work and is it safe?

Benzoyl Peroxide or BPO is a bleach which is thought to work by oxidizing or delivering oxygen to the anaerobic *P. acnes* bacteria in the oil gland and killing it. *P. acnes* is anaerobic (actually aerotolerant) or the type of bacteria which thrives with no oxygen or very low atmospheric oxygen tension and normally protects our skin from invasion by other organisms, such as bacteria and fungus by producing an acid to lower our skin's pH. BPO also causes significant oxidative stress to the surrounding normal tissue causing free radical formation which is how UV light damages skin by interfering with and slowing the skin's healing process and accelerating skin aging. The effects of BPO on skin have been studied in depth and many have reported carcinogenic and pathogenic effects which are toxic to the skin in addition to commonly causing irritation, stinging, burning, extreme dryness and peeling of skin. After all of these years and despite many reports of its potential toxicity, BPO still remains one of the top acne medications in United States. Available in both over-the-counter and prescription formulations, it is a treatment that nearly everyone with acne has tried at some point. Prolonged and high dose use of BPO on acne-burdened skin is likely to cause hypersensitization and significant free radical production and oxidative damage of the skin. Anyone using BPO on regular basis for acne treatment should be treated with regular infusions of anti-oxidant serum to minimize or counter the oxidative damage. I also believe that BPO is much more likely to destroy the accessible *P. acnes* flora in normal pores than penetrating to oxidize the bacteria in the inflamed and encapsulated pustules deep below the keratin layer. I believe that BPO may be one of the more inferior ways to treat acne due to its numerous other side effects. In my practice, we use tailored compounded products containing natural antimicrobials without the potential toxicity of BPO such as tea tree, green tea, rosemary oils and cinnamon bark extract which has the additional benefit of reducing the skin's sebum production, as complements to our intensive hands-on, clearing and disinfection of pustules.

Benzoyl Peroxide has been linked to skin cancer for a number of years and many research journal entries state "benzoyl peroxide is a free radical-generating skin tumor promoting agent." Performing a word search of the words "benzoyl peroxide cancer" in PubMed in the National Library of Medicine produces over 100 articles from medical publications dealing with the research aspects of benzoyl peroxide and cancer. About two-thirds of the research supports linkage between benzoyl peroxide and skin cancer. In 1995, the FDA changed benzoyl peroxide from a Category I (safe) to a Category III (safety is uncertain) ingredient and stated this action (56 FR 37622) was based on new information that raised a safety concern regarding benzoyl peroxide as a tumor promoter in mice. Based on the same information, Over-The-Counter Benzoyl peroxide was banned in EU countries which listed the ingredient as a potential cancer causing agent due to studies in animals showing the repeated application could cause skin tumors.

26. Can your skin get used to acne medications? Is it important to occasionally change your regimen?

I believe that just like many other situations, prolonged exposure of tissue and bacteria to the same products will lead to product fatigue and response will plateau and ultimately decline due to the principle of diminishing returns at which time, the risk for exposure to the product toxicity exceeds its therapeutic benefits and should be stopped. When you start with a regimen to treat active inflamed cystic acne, under optimal conditions, your disease will have some response to treatment and improve; however, the product in the tube or the pill does not make corresponding adjustments to the needs of the improved skin and may no longer be effective or even safe. All products consist of active and inactive chemical ingredients and have therapeutic and toxic profiles. If you continue to use a product without seeing continued benefit, then you are only being exposed to the toxic risks of that product which outweigh the potential benefits. This applies to treating active disease state and not merely maintaining healthy skin clear or antiaging regimen. This is not about acne-prone, a term in which I do not believe, but the acne-burdened skin. Closely observing the skin's response to treatment and continuing to make adjustments to the different components of the treatment while supporting the skin is the underlying basis for our intensive therapeutic approach. Once the skin has been cleared and remains clear during the subsequent maintenance treatments in the office, patient can be transitioned to gentle home-care products without constant changes as the active disease is cleared and maintaining a clear skin becomes much less intensive and more predictable.

It is unlikely, at this stage, for skin that has been restored to clear and healthy to "get used to" or becomes immune to the skin-care products, though the needs of any skin may change over time.

27. Should people with acne-burdened skin use moisturizers?

Yes. but need to be selective and sparing with products. Many people with active acne skip moisturizers because they feel that the more they "dry out" their skin, the better their acne will become. The truth is that some acne patients do have excessive oil production from their sebaceous glands; however, this does not necessarily result in moisturized skin. Under-moisturizing or aggressive cleaning and drying the skin can also result in "rebound" oil production, which makes your skin even oilier. In addition, many acne medications, including over-the-counter spot treatments can be irritating and drying, so it may be necessary to keep acne-burdened skin hydrated. Once patients with acne realize that they need to be moisturizing regularly, they often have questions about the best moisturizer for their skin type. It is important that patients with acne look for moisturizers which are thin, without fragrance and "oil-free". Some of the commercially available moisturizers I recommend to my acne patients are: unscented Cerave ultralight moisturizer, neutrogenia oil-free, ultra-gentle moisturizer and cetaphil Derma control oil control moisturizer. I formulate a special organic moisturizer for patients undergoing my intensive treatments which has a shea butter base and includes oatmeal along with Vitamin E serum to help support the skin with gentle, natural moisture applied to skin while it is still moist after washing. I instruct my patients to avoid the tendency to over moisturize the skin as the skin cannot absorb the moisturizer and needs a better assessment of why it is becoming or feeling so dry. Moisturizers generally cannot penetrate the skin well due to the water-tight keratin barrier. Most moisturizers work as anti-desiccants to keep the skin from losing its natural moisture in the skin layers below the dead, keratin layer. Heavy lotions and creams will likely lead to comedone formation by blocking the skin pores and I do not recommend them. Moisturizers are most effective when applied to skin which is still slightly damp and not completely dry in which case it does not trap the moisture against the skin and will be far less effective.

28. Do at home blue-light devices work as well as in-office treatments?

No. Home blue-light devices are far too weak. The power of the energy required to kill the virulent *P. acnes* bacteria in an encapsulated and inflamed cyst under the skin surface by stimulating the protoporphyrin of the bacteria cannot be achieved by any battery-operated toy. In our office, we use Isolaz, a pneumophototherapy IPL device to disinfect the pustules following extractions as well as Photodynamictherapy with Levulon and blue light which have a much better efficacy in treating the targeted bacteria than any home device. The protective *P. acnes* bacteria that normally lives in our pores is not responsible for developing inflamed cystic acne infections and elimination of this bacteria with injudicious blue-light exposure may disrupt the balance of skin's flora and cause colonization of fungus or opportunistic infection by other competing bacteria. The use of home blue-light devices may also provide a false sense of security and delay more effective and definitive treatment of the cystic acne. Home-care treatments are best for maintenance of clear skin and not treatment of active disease which requires a more intensive and deliberate approach by a physician specializing in the treatment of acne.

29. What is Intensive Acne Care Treatment (I ACT) for inflamed cystic acne?

Our approach to treatment of inflamed cystic acne is the same as treating an abscess and involves weekly extractions, Photopneumatic treatment, additional disinfection of open cysts with chlorhexidine followed by a different chemical peel each week, to stimulate the skin to turn over and push out the next layer of the skin and cysts to the surface for extraction and disinfection the following week. This is complemented by using bespoke compounded products specific to the patient's skin type, acne type and severity to help support and accelerate recovery of the skin to prepare for the next intensive treatment. The treatment is adjusted to skin's dynamic changes on weekly basis with the Isolaz settings and types of filters as well as the type and strength of the chemical peel. The home-care products are also reformulated and adjusted as needed to meet the skin's changing needs as it goes through the series of intensive treatments. Acne is a dynamic disease which changes constantly. Any successful treatment should also be dynamic and prepared to make adjustments to keep up with the skin's changing condition and needs. After all, I believe that a dynamic disease needs an intensive and dynamic treatment to have any hope of clearing the disease. The approach is simple but not easy as it is inconvenient for the patient and intensive, requiring a deliberate, hands-on treatment method, not magic. I believe treating inflamed cystic acne with lotions, potions, pills and prayers is a magical and mystical approach with heavy reliance on faith more than scientific evidence. Inflamed, cystic acne is an abscess (i.e. a surgical infection), which requires surgical treatment to open, drain and disinfect to allow the tissue to heal and restore health. The key is an evidence-based, deliberate treatment method based on sound and consistent philosophy of the disease to guide the treatment through precise and targeted procedures and direct observation of the infection being cleared layer by skin layer.

30. How are antibiotics used to treat acne?

Antibiotics are frequently over-used or abused in the mainstream treatment of acne despite evidence that prolonged use of systemic antibiotics is not effective against the bacteria causing inflamed cystic acne and likely hazardous to the individual's as well as the general public's health. Systemic antibiotics are not a treatment of choice for surgical infections such as an abscess which is encapsulated and inflamed. The pill is expected to survive salivary enzymes, gastric acid, bile salt, intestinal enzymes, liver processing, going through 6 liters of blood as it is being pumped through heart and lung just to deliver very small amount of the remaining active ingredient into the inflamed cyst on the skin. It is not practical or logical to expect to clear a pustule which is superficial and accessible to simple drainage and disinfection without causing significant morbidity or any damage to the rest of the body as oral antibiotics do with prolonged use. No doctor or dentist treats an abscess with oral or topical antibiotics or other chemicals, as it is well established that an abscess must be opened, drained and disinfected to clear. The inflamed cystic eruptions on the skin are no different just because someone decides to call them "acne". The principle of an abscess being a surgical infection which requires surgical treatment remains as the guiding directive of my approach to treating this type of acne. During the course of treatment, we often have a purge of the cystic acne, especially in the early stages of the intensive treatment. This is the only time I am inclined to use a short course of oral antibiotics for up to 2-weeks, to minimize spread and inflammation of the surrounding skin. Prolonged or indefinite use of antibiotics is ill-advised and inconsiderate with no basis in evidence; especially, as there is growing evidence of the dangers of antibiotic-resistant bacteria to the public health.

31. Are topical antibiotics effective against inflamed cystic acne?

Not in my experience. The most common topical antibiotic used in dermatology today for the treatment of acne is clindamycin which may be combined with Benzoyl Peroxide or tretinoin. Other topical antibiotics in use today for treatment of acne are Erythromycin and Dapsone. Although more targeted to the acne location with less systemic risks, topical antibiotics are unlikely to penetrated through inflamed walls of an abscess to clear and disinfect it. Topical antibiotics are best used for treatment of open wound infections such as abrasions, not enclosed and encapsulated infections such as abscess. The only circumstance where I have found topical antibiotic to be useful is the use of metronidazole gel to treat suspected or confirmed Rosacea.

32. What are the side effects of oral antibiotics?

All oral antibiotics have side effects, which is why they should be used judiciously, deliberately and sparingly. Placing an individual on prolonged, indefinite or repeated courses of antibiotics is potentially very harmful to the individual as well as the public at large. Systemic antibiotics will decimate the bacteria that form our natural flora and protect us from parasitic microorganisms, balance the pH to allow optimal function of enzymes as well as allowing us to breakdown and digest nutrients through our intestinal tract. Prolonged use of antibiotics not only destroys the protective bacteria, it may lead to the formation of drug-resistant strains of virulent or pathogenic bacteria. Ultimately the important consideration before starting any patient on antibiotics, especially for acne is the objective and the end game. Is the objective suppression of the inflamed cystic eruptions or definitive clearance? What do you do if after starting the antibiotics, the acute inflammation clears? Do you stop or continue? If you continue, how do you know it's still necessary? If you stop and inflammatory cysts erupt again, do you go back on the antibiotics, the same or different, stronger dose, for how long this time? You cannot engage in this type of chemical warfare against a much better positioned and entrenched organism without having a definitive and deliberate plan of action with well-articulated definition of success and failure and strategies to terminate, pivot or make small adjustments and what the alternate approach would be in case of setback or lack of response. It is unreasonable to expose an individual to the significant risks of prolonged and random antibiotic use for the treatment of inflamed cystic acne when the disease is surgical and not mystical, magical or medical. We normally go out of our way to buy organic food because it was not contaminated with antibiotics and hormones but then we are placed on massive doses of both of these potentially harmful drugs to treat acne, a disease which is not a threat to limb or life. That is unreasonable.

I believe we need to save the use of antibiotics for acute medical infections in short bursts to maintain bacterial sensitivity and susceptibility to common antibiotics in the future and treat surgical infections, surgically. Physicians have learned not to keep prescribing antibiotics for ear infections, coughs or sore throats unless there is a specific bacterial infection and even then, if it seems to be recurring, the patients are referred to a surgeon for placement of tubes to ventilate the middle ear or removal of the tonsils and the adenoids as a much more definitive treatment to minimize further use of antibiotics. Why have we not learned this lesson with acne? I believe acne is the major reason for prolonged, unnecessary and ineffective antibiotics use in the developed nations, especially in the United States and western Europe. This is unreasonable and counter to good public health policy.

33. How long does it take to see results from prescription medications?

In my experience, the results of topical or systemic chemicals on acne are unpredictable, sporadic and temporary. The encapsulated and inflamed pustule is generally not permeable or responsive to chemicals applied through the waxy layer of the skin or the blood that feeds the skin. Generally, if these medications do reduce the acne inflammation it's mainly through suppression of inflammation, not elimination of infection. Ultimately, for a disease to be managed through suppression, it will require long-term use of the suppressants and continued sensitivity to the suppressant. It is not unusual to have breakthroughs of the disease on suppressive treatment as the levels of the active ingredients fluctuate and body's response to the chemicals changes under different conditions. This is how acne becomes transformed from an acute infection into a chronic medical disease requiring prolonged chemotherapy to keep the disease in remission. As we have seen with many other disease processes, remission does not mean eradication. Frequently, once the suppressive chemotherapy is stopped, because the individual wants to or needs to, the disease that re-emerges is much more fulminant partly because the host's immune response remains impaired or suppressed, causing a more aggressive and extensive disease.

34. Are there risks with prolonged oral antibiotics related to taking oral birth control?

Yes, as oral birth control pills, which are frequently prescribed for treatment of acne in women, deliver hormones such as estrogen and especially progesterone to the blood stream that are bound by proteins such as albumin in the blood. The bioavailability of these hormones and thus their effectiveness is directly related to the level of bound vs. free hormones. Antibiotics frequently displace or alter the protein binding of hormones and significantly alter their bioavailability and their efficacy or potency. Thus, reliance of oral birth controls for birth control or suppression of inflammatory skin eruptions becomes unpredictable and risky. In my practice, I do not recommend oral birth control for acne suppression and I only use oral antibiotics in short bursts of no more than 2-weeks which limits these risks.

35. Can oral antibiotics make me more sensitive to sun?

Yes, many oral antibiotics are light-sensitizing, meaning that you are more likely to get sunburned if you are taking them. Drugs in the Tetracycline class, such as Doxycycline and minocycline are especially light-sensitizing as compared to many other antibiotics commonly used in the treatment of acne. This means it is very important to practice strict sun avoid or physical protection when on these medication.

36. Will being on an oral antibiotic make me resistant to this antibiotic if I need it in the future?

Possibly, since the antibiotic is to treat pathogenic bacteria and there is strong evidence that the bacteria become resistant to the antibiotics with frequent or prolonged exposure. The individual may suffer from other side effects of the antibiotics having to do most commonly with injury to liver function and intestinal flora. It is well established in the medical literature that the promiscuous use of antibiotics does lead to widespread bacterial resistance which may well make it much more difficult to treat infections with our current antibiotics in the future.

37. What is Retin-A?

Retin-A is a brand name of tretinoin, an example of topical retinoid. Retinoids are Vitamin A derivatives which are used to accelerate skin cell turn-over and help with anti-aging support of the skin such as reducing fine wrinkles. In my experience, retinoids do not help in treating inflammation nor are they useful in resolution or prevention of pustules. If one is to believe that comedones start with retention hyperkeratosis which is blockage of the pilosebaceous pore with dead skin cell, then accelerating the turn-over and shedding of the skin would not only not help reduce comedones but theoretically worsen it. Topical retinoid application will also make the skin more sensitive in general and more specifically to sun exposure. Use of topical retinoids will likely accelerate and potentiate more cystic eruptions to the surface of the skin; however, if these eruptions are not manually cleared and disinfected, then they will likely persist while causing inflammatory damage to the skin. Also, prolonged use of topical retinoids is known to dry the skin which further sensitizes and dysregulates the skin's normal oil production and response to environmental irritants or injury. Long-term use of topical retinoids can cause excessive redness and even peeling. If irritation occurs after applying a retinoid, (this is called "retinoid dermatitis"), stop using the medication for a few days and as the skin is healing you may apply over-the-counter hydrocortisone twice daily for up to five days and use as a gentle moisturizer. I do not recommend restarting retinoids once your skin heals.

38. Are acne treatments anti-aging?

Some of the conventional topical treatments such as Alpha or Beta Hydroxy acids and retinoids may have anti-aging effects. However, others such as Benzoyl Peroxide will likely age the skin through oxidative stress similar to sun exposure. Isotretinoin's anti-aging effect is attributed to potential collagen stimulation as a result of increased skin cell turnover. However, collagen which contributes to skin elasticity is mostly produced by fibroblast cells which live in the deeper dermis layer and thus unlikely to stimulate any meaningful collagen synthesis. As a complement to surgical extraction, Light-based approach to treatment of inflamed, cystic acne using Intense Pulsed Blue and Red light and Photodynamic therapy is highly effective against the bacterial cause of acne while presenting very low risk to the surrounding tissue and no risk to the rest of the body and can be used as needed for as long as needed without selecting for resistant strains of bacteria as antibiotics do or cause tissue damage as many topicals do. Phototherapy using an IPL has also long been an effective and safe tool for skin restoration and of anti-aging. Although sunscreen is protective of the oxidative effects of the Sun's Ultraviolet rays in an intact, normal and healthy skin, it is potentially toxic and damaging in a brittle, sensitive and compromised acne-burdened and inflamed skin. Sun protection through use of effective physical barriers and sun avoidance are key to enhancing the anti-aging effects of Phototherapy or chemical peels and must be practiced diligently along with liberal use of oil-free, fragrance-free and Paraben-free moisturizers as needed.

39. What is Accutane?

Accutane as a brand name is no longer made in the U.S.; however, Oral Isotretinoin, the generic drug is available and frequently prescribed for acne. Isotretinoin, which is a synthetic Vitamin A derivative, was created and used as a chemotherapeutic agent to treat severe nodulocystic acne as well as various types of cancer. Isotretinoin is a serious drug with potentially serious health risks and it should not be prescribed for the common acne or localized cystic acne. In my opinion, the only circumstances under which this drug should be prescribed is for treatment of Acne Conglobata or Fulminans and in rare cases where the inflamed nodulocystic acne has not responded to intensive procedural approach. The drug is a differentiating agent which interferes with oil gland function leading to significant reduction or cessation of oil production and skin turnover and regeneration. It is likely that its effect on reducing the inflammation of acne is through suppression of the individual's immune response and not through eradication of the underlying cause of the inflammation, the infection. In my opinion, Isotretinoin is a toxic and potentially teratogenic drug with a black-box label by the FDA which should only be prescribed for treatment of severe and widespread or deforming nodulocystic eruptions.

Here is a brief history of Accutane, from the time it was approved in 1982 to the present day.

1982 The FDA approves Hoffmann-La Roche's Accutane (isotretinoin), a prescription medication for use in treating severe acne that is unresponsive to conventional therapies. The FDA gives Accutane the Category X pregnancy rating, which means it's contraindicated during pregnancy.

1984 The FDA requires a "black-box" warning for Accutane, citing the risk for fetal deformity.

1998 Several medical studies cite a possible link between depression and Accutane use. The FDA issues a warning to physicians, and Accutane warning labels in the US are updated to include a possible risk of adverse psychiatric effects, including depression, psychosis, suicidal ideation and suicide.

1989 The FDA mandates the implementation of the Accutane Pregnancy Prevention Program.

2000 The FDA and Accutane manufacturer Hoffmann-La Roche agree to link a negative pregnancy test with each monthly prescription of Accutane.

2001 A Medication Guide is approved to provide more plain language information about Accutane's side effects. It is to be distributed by pharmacists to Accutane patients. The FDA also establishes an online Accutane Drug Information web page. Hoffmann-La Roche approves the use of the SMART (System to Manage Accutane Related Teratogenicity) program for pregnancy prevention. Key elements include patient-informed consent, pregnancy testing and contraception use.

2002 The FDA becomes aware through the Adverse Event Reporting System of 173 reports of suicide associated with Accutane treatment worldwide. The FDA requires Hoffmann-La Roche to begin submitting quarterly summaries of side effects. By August 2002, the summaries include roughly 6,000 additional reports of psychiatric adverse events, such as depression and suicidal thoughts. The FDA begins to collaborate with the National Institute of Mental Health to address the need for more independent research and holds a workshop to discuss basic scientific research into the effects of retinoids on the central nervous system. Hoffmann-La Roche starts including a Medication Guide in the Accutane blister pack. The guide will later become part of the iPLEDGE program. Hoffmann-La Roche's original patent for Accutane expires. In the first 20 years of Accutane use, the FDA Adverse Event Reporting System contains almost 23,000 reports for Accutane, mostly from the US. The 5 most frequent reactions are alopecia (hair loss), depression, headache, dry skin and induced abortion to purposely end a pregnancy conceived while taking Accutane. The FDA approves the first generic version of isotretinoin called Amnesteem.

2002-2003 Generic isotretinoin versions of Amnesteem, Sotret and Claravis each propose a separate pregnancy-risk program to avoid pregnancy while taking the drug.

2003 Hoffmann-La Roche and other isotretinoin drug manufacturers agree to work together on the need for a single pregnancy prevention program. Accutane use starts to decline from 284,925 (2000) to 128,936 (2003) for men and from 278,252 (2000) to 128,973 (2003) for women, according to a Hoffmann-La Roche presentation to the FDA Advisory Committee.

2004 The FDA Joint Advisory Committee recommends a single, required, stronger risk management plan for all marketed isotretinoin products. The plan links isotretinoin prescriptions with pregnancy testing to reduce the chance of a pregnancy during treatment.

2005 The FDA issues an alert for Accutane and all generic isotretinoin, advising doctors to monitor patients for suicidal thoughts or actions. Wholesalers, pharmacies and prescribers begin registering for the iPLEDGE Program in September 2005. Patients begin registering for the program on December 30, 2005.

2006 In March, iPLEDGE pharmacies are required to obtain iPLEDGE system authorization before filling an Accutane or isotretinoin prescription. (Both patients and prescribers must prove they are registered with iPLEDGE.) Women of childbearing age are required to provide their doctors with a current negative pregnancy test result each month before receiving a prescription.

2007 The FDA warns about purchasing Accutane or generic isotretinoin versions online. The first case alleging that Accutane causes inflammatory bowel disease (IBD) results in a $2.6 million award. In October, a jury awards another plaintiff $7 million for a case involving IBD.

2008 A New Jersey Superior Court jury awards $10.5 million in a case, one of 425 against Hoffmann-La Roche, alleging the drug causes IBD. (The judgment will be reversed in 2010.)

2009 Hoffmann-La Roche voluntarily removes Accutane from the market, citing competition from generic isotretinoin versions.

2010 The American Academy of Dermatology (AAD) issues an updated position statement on the use of isotretinoin. It claims that, according to published scientific studies, there is no direct causal relationship between isotretinoin and IBD and psychiatric disturbances. The AAD calls for the need for patient monitoring and more scientific testing on the topic. In February, a jury awards Andrew McCarrell $25 million, the largest Accutane award to date. McCarrell claims he developed IBD years after taking Accutane. (This judgment will be upheld in 2011.)

2012 In June, a New Jersey Superior Court orders Hoffmann-La Roche to pay $18 million in compensatory damages to 2 Accutane users who developed ulcerative colitis. The court found in Hoffmann-La Roche's favor in 2 other cases.

2013 U.S. District Court dismissed 40 Accutane lawsuits when plaintiffs failed to meet court deadlines to produce an expert witness.

2014 Hoffmann-La Roche wins a reversal of a $2 million Accutane trial verdict. A former Accutane user had blamed the drug for her IBD — a condition she had years prior to taking Accutane. Hoffmann-La Roche continues to sell isotretinoin under the name Roaccutane in other countries. Other governments are still reviewing claims of psychiatric adverse events including suicide linked to Roaccutane use.

2015 A New Jersey appeals court reversed Andrew McCarrell's $25.2 million jury verdict against Roche (see above), ruling that McCarrell waited too long to bring the case. McCarrell will appeal, according to one of his lawyers.

2017 N.J. Supreme Court reinstates $25M verdict in Accutane case

2018 N.J. Supreme Court ended all product liability lawsuits in MCL 271.

FREQUENTLY ASKED QUESTIONS

40. Is Accutane safe?

When properly monitored, and prescribed by an experienced medical professional to treat severe, inflamed, nodulocystic acne, Accutane (i.e. Isotretinoin) can be a safe and effective medication just as any chemotherapy drug used in an attempt to treat a life-threatening disease. However, none of the acne cases are life-threatening and the overwhelming majority are not severe enough to warrant the short and long-term risks associated with this drug.

41. Is Accutane safe for teenagers?

Teenagers with severe nodulocystic acne that have not responded to hands-on procedural treatments may be appropriate candidates for Accutane therapy. Accutane has many potential side effects but when properly managed, can be a safe and effective medication. Accutane, in addition to many of the well-known side-effects, may be inappropriate for young individuals due to stunting growth by causing premature epiphyseal fusion (growth plate) of the long bones and decrease cartilage formation. It is also inappropriate for young individuals who spend a great deal of time outdoors during the day exposed to sun due to photosensitization of skin by Isotretinoin. In addition to Isotretinoin, the young female will be started on oral birth control which may additionally disrupt or dysregulate the endocrine system. However, many teenagers do very well with procedural and light-based treatments for acne avoiding the potential long-term side effects of Isotretinoin chemotherapy with better treatment compliance.

42. What is the most common side effect of Accutane?

The most common side effect of Accutane is excessive dryness of the skin and lips, which is found in the majority of patients. Patients may find that their lips, mouth, eyes and skin are very dry. Moisturizing by frequent application of topicals is often inadequate, which may lead to non-compliance and ultimate failure of treatment. Other, less common but not rare side effects include worsening depression, gastrointestinal and liver damage.

43. How long does it take for Accutane to clear the system?

The half-life of Accutane in your body is 18-20 hours so by 2 weeks, it is completely out of your system. This is why women are advised by their dermatologist that they can get pregnant 1 month after their last Accutane dose as the assumption is that there is no actual Accutane left circulating in the body at that time. However, there is no evidence that a few of the existing eggs in the woman's body at the time of Isotretinoin administration were not permanently damaged and may lead to a longer teratogenic effect if one of the damaged eggs is fertilized in the future. In terms of Accutane skin effects, this can last longer than the medication half-life itself. Due to significant thinning of the epidermis from Accutane, the risk of skin injury and delayed healing is high and it takes 6-12 months for skin to thicken enough to recover properly from injury from physical trauma, chemical peels and laser. Symptoms and side-effects also persists for months as the biological effects of Accutane take a lot longer to reverse even though the toxic metabolites of Accutane are out of the system.

44. What should I look for in skin care product and makeup formulations if I have acne?

The critical product is the foundation or the concealer which can potentially cause the most stress on the skin. It is best to select a breathable formulation which can also help keep the oil glands from clogging. The brand I recommend to my patients is the medicated Oxygenetix formulation which offers numerous shades to best match the tone. Otherwise, I would advise that any enhancing makeup being applied on top of the foundation or concealer have as few ingredients as possible with no fragrance and preferably powder-based, mineral formulations. Most liquid makeup requires exposure to significant heat to emulsify which causes denaturation of the components and formation of toxic byproduct and usually requires preservatives which can further injure the brittle and compromised acne-burdened skin. Most products which have water as a main ingredient require preservatives to prevent microbial contamination; however, remain a great reservoir and breeding ground for bacteria which can then colonize or infect the skin after repeated applications. I also recommend that any paste or liquid-based product being used on the skin be packed in tubes or pumps to avoid high risk of contamination by repeated placement of finger or an applicator into the product. If using products in open jars, I recommend storing them in a refrigerator or at room temperature. Avoid storing in the bathroom where they may be exposed to heat and humidity which will increase the likelihood of microbial contamination and more rapid disintegration and denaturation.

45. Does diet cause acne?

We have always been told that "we are what we eat" as certain foods are known to contribute to flare ups; however, the relationship between diet and acne is highly controversial. Compelling evidence shows that high glycemic load diets may exacerbate acne. Dairy ingestion appears to be weakly associated with acne and the roles of omega-3 fatty acids, dietary fiber, antioxidants, vitamin A, zinc and iodine remain to be elucidated. Numerous studies have revealed that clinical imbalances of specific essential fatty acids are associated with a variety of skin problems. Hence dry, itchy, scaly skin is a hallmark sign of fatty acid deficiency and Linoleic fatty acid has been shown to be deficient in the sebum of acne-burdened individuals. In the body, linoleic acid is converted to arachidonic acid, a precursor to pro-inflammatory compounds that can have detrimental effects on health. Understanding the importance of these "side-effects" of consuming linoleic acid has led to the widely-adopted approach of countering these Omega-6 pro-inflammatory fatty acids with Omega-3 fatty acids. Currently the best evidence-based recommendation with regards to diet in individuals suffering from inflammatory acne is to adopt a low glycemic index diet, high in Omega 3 fatty acids and various fruits and vegetables high in antioxidants and various vitamins along with 6-8 glasses of water daily for proper hydration based on level of activity. Although a healthy diet may reduce the extent of inflammation, diet does not cause inflamed cystic acne and change in diet will not clear acne without intensive treatment, just as change in diet and lifestyle will not clear a dental infection. Clearing acne and achieving sustainable, long-term skin health requires diet and life-style modifications only as a complement to intensive hands-on treatment under the care of a physician specializing in acne treatment, not in place of.

Estheticians are not dieticians. Dieticians have degrees in dietetics, the science of nutrition. In most states, dieticians are licensed and regulated. Persons who are not licensed or registered dieticians or physicians are not qualified to give advice on nutrition. Estheticians are not trained in nutrition to recommend dietary changes for their clients. Clients may have medical conditions, such as diabetes or high blood pressure that can be negatively effected by misinformation and unqualified advice. This is particularly true in the treatment of acne in salons and spas.

46. Does chocolate cause acne?

I believe that cystic acne is an opportunistic infection and it is not caused by food. The better question is whether chocolate can worsen existing acne. There is evidence that chocolate milk may have more direct association with worsening of acne rather than dark chocolate as dark chocolate is higher in anti-oxidants whereas, milk chocolate contains much more refined carbohydrates high in glycemic index which is known to increase inflammation by raising the Insulin level and worsen any inflammatory skin condition including cystic acne.

FREQUENTLY ASKED QUESTIONS

47. Does being over-weight contribute to worsening acne?

While an unhealthy diet may not be a direct cause of acne formation or major reason for increasing acne breakouts, it turns out obesity is associated with more potential to develop acne in teens, especially young women. No direct cause and effect relationship has been proposed; however, the most likely explanation is creation of metabolic syndrome with elevated blood sugars, increase in insulin production as well as dysregulation and derangement of estrogen and androgen production which modulate the individual's immune response to the bacterial infection.

48. Is it true that sugar and dairy will make breakouts worse?

Pro-inflammatory foods such as carbohydrates and sugars which cause increase in glycemia or blood sugar content, are likely to make inflamed cystic acne worse but do not cause it. It is also not clear with regards to mild consumption, if it is the lactose sugar or much less likely, growth hormones which are administered to cattle to enhance milk production that may persist in sufficient level in pasteurized, commercial milk to cause androgenic stimulation of sebaceous glands. I believe that individuals who are struggling with inflamed cystic acne eruptions are well served by reducing their sugar intake which includes fructose and lactose and not just sucrose.

Sugar and dairy do not cause acne. However, recent studies have suggested that sugar and dairy may influence the extent or severity of inflammation associated with pustular acne. Interestingly, in countries that consume a low glycemic and low dairy diet, inflammatory acne is much less common. Of course, there are other factors that may come into play, but this suggests that sugar and milk may play a role in exacerbating inflammation.

Consumption of dairy may contribute to inflammation by its effect on hormone signaling. Milk contains IGF-1, an insulin-like growth hormone which helps young bodies develop necessary tissues. Increased levels of IGF-1 result in increased skin cell and oil production which may contribute to retention hyperkeratosis and clogging of the pores as well as stimulation of bacteria infecting the oil glands which lead to worsening of acne.

49. What is the connection between Peanut butter and acne?

Peanut butter has a high fat content with two tablespoons containing 16g of fat, nearly 50% of which is monounsaturated and 30% polyunsaturated. A healthy ratio of omega 3 to 6 is needed to avoid exuberant inflammation (somewhere in the region of 1:1 to 1:4). The fats in peanut butter are omega-6 fats, most of which is LA (linoleic acid), which the body can convert to AA (arachidonic acid), which is what triggers inflammation. In addition to the omega-6 fats (arachidonic acid) in peanut butter triggering inflammation, they are highly unstable and easily react with heat and oxygen in the body, triggering a chain-reaction of peroxidized fatty acids, which eventually break down into toxins like malondialdehyde (MDA) that can damage the fundamental structures of basically any cell in your body.

The body better regulates the extent of inflammation if the omega 3/6 ratio is at the ideal level. Peanut butter, being so high in omega-6, can very easily upset the delicate balance between omega 3 and 6. The body uses omega-6 fats to produce cytokines and prostaglandins, which start inflammation, signaling immune cells to rush in and heal the injury and if there is too much omega-6 fat in the body (by eating foods like peanut butter), the body has trouble stopping inflammation. That's because omega-3s are required to halt inflammation. (Specifically, DHA.) Remember, omega-6s start inflammation, omega-3s stop it. The average American, for example, has more like a 20:1 ratio of omega-6:3 rather than the ideal 1:1 to 4:1 which is likely to cause what's called systemic inflammation. That is, when the body is under a more-or-less constant state of low-grade inflammation., causing red, swollen, painful pimples that stick around for a long time!

Secondly, consumption of large amount of omega-6 fats tends to promote what's called "Small Intestinal Bacterial Overgrowth" (SIBO). That's where the small intestine gets colonized by a ton of bad bacteria. It's not supposed to have many bacteria (compared to the colon / large intestine), but in SIBO things get way out of hand. SIBO can worsen acne, because all those bacteria tend to produce toxins which not only cause increase generalized inflammation, compromise the immune system but also cause significant intestinal inflammation, malabsorption and vitamin (antioxidant) deficiency. Peanut butter, like all other grains and legumes, contain a protein called agglutinin which also cause digestive problems by increasing intestinal permeability ("leaky gut") resulting in food particles passing through into the blood stream, triggering an autoimmune response, food allergies and systemic inflammation all of which will make response to acne worse.

Thirdly, peanut butter, along with corn, are the main sources of aflatoxin, which is a toxin created by molds (fungi) of the Aspergillus genus. While a direct link to acne has not been established, aflatoxin is a known contributor to liver cancer, kidney cancer, malnutrition, and birth defects. Peanut butter is one of the better ways to consume peanuts. The peanut-butter-making process in commercial brands reduces aflatoxin by 89% although the grind-it-yourself peanut butter in natural food stores has the most aflatoxin.

Lastly, the most insidious problem with peanut butter is that it's almost always packed with sugar and gluten. The majority of commercial peanut butter is made with hydrogenated oils and sugar. The hydrogenated oils keep the fat from separating, and the sugar, obviously, makes it sweet. Hydrogenated oils are bad for acne for the same reason described above, and sugar will increase insulin production, increased inflammation, glycation, and a compromised immune system.

50. Can caffeine worsen acne breakouts?

One of the things it does is to magnify our stress response. The scientific term is that it induces a state of "hyperadrenalism", making the adrenal glands pump out excessive hormones such as stress hormones which cause cortisone release, increase in inflammation, release of insulin and additional hormonal imbalance which will compromise the immune response and increase the risk of infection such as acne and subsequently, a deranged inflammatory response, leading to exaggerated and prolonged redness and pain.

51. Does a high-glucose diet play a part in acne breakouts?

There is no evidence that diet causes acne as it is an infection; however, a high glycemic index diet can compromise the immune system and make the skin more susceptible to an infection and cause a more exaggerated inflammatory response to low grade infections, resulting in pustules that are likely to cause scars. Empirically, there is evidence that a low-carbohydrate, low-glycemic diet might in fact help reduce inflammation associated with acne. This type of management or modulation of inflammation does not happen overnight and will require months of disciplined adherence to the diet. Such a diet along with intensive, hands-on acne treatment will create conditions where a clear and healthy skin is much more sustainable long-term than constant use of topical or system chemicals to manage acne.

Some examples of high-glycemic foods include Foods that are the processed, simple carbohydrates such as white bread products, cookies, candy, white rice, white potatoes and breakfast cereals. When a food registers high on the GI. It means that its carbohydrates break down quickly and release glucose into bloodstream at a faster pace than other food.

52. Does drinking milk affect my acne?

Despite reports suggesting a small association of increase in acne eruptions with milk consumption, no cause and effect or actual mechanism of action has been established. The fact is that Lactose is a sugar and consumption of any sugars will lead to increase in inflammation as previously discussed. The suggestion that hormones injected into cows to increase their milk production somehow survive various processes such as pasteurization to cause hormonal derangement in the consumer as the cause of acne is not factual. Bovine growth hormone (bGH, also called bovine somatotropin, bST) is made from amino acids, just like any other protein we eat and digest. There are no studies that indicate that growth hormone from milk should be able to survive our digestion or that fragments from this digestion has any biological activity. In fact, nothing suggests that growth hormone from cows even have an effect on our own human growth hormone receptors. But even if this was the case – even if bGH was biologically active in humans – the amount of growth hormone in cow's milk is miniscule, and 85-90% of it is destroyed during the heat treatment milk goes through during production. The tiny amount that is left is in all likelihood readily digested in the intestine and absorbed as amino acids, as is the case with any other dietary protein. Additionally, **milk contains the same amount of IGF-1 as your own saliva**. There are no studies suggesting that intake of IGF-1 cow's milk has any discernible biological activity in humans.

53. Are there medications that can help better control systemic inflammation caused by elevated blood sugar?

Metformin is one of the oldest and most studied drugs available in the United States. Other names for metformin include Glucophage, Glucophage XR, glumetza, and fortamet. Metformin works as an insulin-sensitizer to reduce production of glucose. Metformin lowers blood glucose and insulin levels by suppressing the liver's production of glucose, increasing the sensitivity of liver, muscle, fat, and cells to the insulin body makes and decreasing the absorption of carbohydrates consumed. I have occasionally used metformin as an adjunct in treatment of moderate-to-severe acne, especially in women with or without a confirmed diagnosis of Poly Cystic Ovarian Syndrome (PCOS) or overweight males with good results.

Although it's not labeled for use in women with PCOS, metformin is one of the most common medications used to manage the condition. Metformin has been studied in girls as young as 8 years of age, with some researchers recommending it to prevent the onset of PCOS. The average dose of metformin I recommend for women with PCOS is 1,500 mg to 2,000 mg daily and 500 to 1000 in those without a confirmed diagnosis of PCOS and no history of hypoglycemic episodes with otherwise average diets.

54. Can oral contraceptive pills help to treat adult acne?

A few oral contraceptive pills, such as Yaz and Yasmin, have FDA indication for the treatment of acne, though by enlarge, flooding the body with significant amount of synthetic hormones to control acne through creating a significant hormonal imbalance is not a good idea and has many other potential risks to the rest of the body such as liver damage and potential increased risk of venous thromboembolism. Oral contraceptives simulate pregnancy and are beneficial for oily skin in that they result in a decrease in ovarian and adrenal androgens and increase sex hormone-binding globulin, which limits free testosterone. Ultimately, even if oral birth control helps reduce the extent of inflammatory acne eruptions, it is only working as-long-as you continue to take it and at some point, all women will either want to or need to discontinue this type of hormonal manipulation of their body and often acne which was being hormonally suppressed, may rebound with intensity. I have found that the best and most effective ways to treat acne in women in their childbearing years are often through intensive, hands-on treatment utilizing extractions, light therapy, cortisone injection,

FREQUENTLY ASKED QUESTIONS

and prescription oral medications such as Spironolactone and Metformin and topical medications.

55. How do you treat increase in testosterone in men and women with inflammatory cystic acne?

If a hyperandrogen state is thought to be contributing to the severity of inflammatory response to acne, I have used oral Antiandrogens in both men and women to reduce the effects of testosterone on skin as a complement to procedural, intensive treatments until inflamed cystic acne and pustules resolve. Androgens, particularly 5α- dihydrotestosterone (dHt), play a major role in the differentiation and proliferation of sebaceous glands as well as sebum production and proliferation. Spironolactone has been shown to directly reduce sebum production when dosed 50 to 200mg daily. In addition to being an aldosterone antagonist, spironolactone also functions as an androgen receptor blocker and an inhibitor of 5α-reductase. Similarly, in men, I have successfully and safely used Finasteride as an antiandrogen to inhibit 5 alpha-reductase and reduce dHt as an adjunct for treatment of inflamed pustular acne.

56. Does LED light help to treat adult acne?

Red and blue LED lights in the doctor's office can be used to maintain clear skin as penetration of the LED rays into the skin is minimal. Red light reduces inflammation and blue LED light kills *P. acnes* bacteria. There is no downtime after the LED treatment. However, when LED treatments are combined with photosensitizing chemicals such as levulonic acid, the PhotoDynamic Therapy (PDT) has a potential to cause dramatic reduction of inflammatory cystic acne with elimination of the bacterial infection as well as reduction of oil production.

57. What is a cortisone injection and should I be getting them?

Cortisone injections are an in-office procedure, administered by a doctor and a good option for those who need to promptly put down an acute inflamed acne eruption. Cortisone injections contain a low concentration of an anti-inflammatory medication called Triamcinolone, which is a corticosteroid medication, a catabolic steroid unlike testosterone which is anabolic. It is injected right into the inflamed pustule. I frequently combine it with clindamycin antibiotic solution and keep the steroid concentration between 0.1-0.15 mg to reduce the risk of causing indentation or loss of pigmentation at the site of injection. Over the next 24-48 hours, the anti-inflammatory effects of Triamcinolone take effect and the acne lesion will flatten out. Most inflammatory acne lesions can be treated with a cortisone injection on an emergency basis; however, it should not be used as a regular treatment for persistent, recurrent or extensive acne. In my practice, I also have successfully used injection of non-steroidal anti-inflammatory drug, Ketorolac to treat inflamed nodulocystic acne eruptions without the risk of collagen atrophy and skin depression at the site of injection, which is not an uncommon risk of cortisone injection.

58. What is acne extraction?

During a session of medical extractions, a skin care provider may heat your skin for a few minutes to bring to surface and soften the cysts or abscesses. The provider will then sharply open each abscess which has broken through the surface with a sharp lancet and then evacuate the contents of the abscess followed by disinfection using Isolaz to deliver intense blue bactericidal light into the open cysts followed by scrubbing with a chemical disinfectant such as Chlorhexidine gluconate.

Extractions are critical in the definitive treatment of inflamed nodulocystic acne since only surgical drainage and disinfection has always been the standard of care for any skin abscess. The extractions are usually performed in conjunction with other in-office treatments such as Isolaz Photopneumatic therapy to further disinfect the open abscess as well as reduce the acute inflammation by delivering intense blue and red light onto and into the lesions.

My intensive approach to cystic acne treatment often combines weekly extraction, evacuation and disinfection of the inflamed skin abscesses with chemical peels, in order to increase skin turnover and force a purge of the deeper cysts and nodules. Additionally, as an adjunct to the hands-on treatments, I compound and provide individualized skin-care products along with select prescriptions to support the skin and promote faster recovery between the intensive treatments. Patients may notice some redness, dryness and flaking of the treated area after a treatment, but may apply specialized makeup if desired after at least 4 hours. We also recommend applying a cold compress to the face after every in-office treatment as well as anytime when the skin feels inflamed and avoid heat or steam which will worsen inflammation. Most patients are able to resume professional or social activities immediately following the treatment although they are advised to refrain from strenuous physical activity and sweating for at least 4 hours to minimize inflammation of the traumatized treatment area.

59. Do you recommend seeing an esthetician for extractions of inflamed cysts?

No, as mere extraction of the abscess is insufficient and likely harmful without proper disinfection and skin support. However, comedonal extractions by medically unsupervised estheticians is low risk if the goal is to merely clear clogged pores in blackheads and whiteheads without any inflamed pustules. Generally, the depth of penetration into the dermis required to drain a pustule is outside the scope of practice of aestheticians as the licensing boards have restricted the cosmetologist to work only on dead tissue such as nails, hair and keratin. Since acne originates much deeper than the keratin layer, it is in living tissue and thus outside the scope of a medically unsupervised aesthetician or cosmetologist. By definition. Since pus and blood only exist in living tissue, any procedures that result in release of pus or blood are considered practice of medicine and should not be performed in a salon or spa, even "medspa" since there is rarely a doctor on site to provide proper diagnosis and treatment plan, let alone perform the procedure.

It is also important to recognize that not all skin bumps are acne and effective treatment of any disease or condition is contingent on proper initial diagnosis which is the cornerstone of practice of medicine and should be done by a qualified physician specializing in diagnosis and treatment of acne. If a dangerous lesion is mistaken for acne by a medically unsupervised aesthetician, there may be a critical delay in diagnosis and timely implementation of the definitive treatment that may lead to significant and avoidable morbidity.

60. What is the difference in "popping" the pustule versus medical extraction?

First, popping pustules or zits is never a good idea; whether performed by the acne-burdened individual or the cosmetologist using her fingers which lead to uncontrolled rupture of the cyst and not a careful and deliberate extraction of the pus through a small, controlled opening on the cyst surface. Popping can lead to spread of infection internally, further breakouts, increased inflammation, scars and irreparable damage. Plus, the chances of fully removing the pus and disinfecting the cyst without proper medical tools is very low.

61. Does Intense Pulsed Light (IPL) help active acne?

Intense pulsed light (IPL) has been shown to help both inflamed cystic acne in conjunction with extractions and the reactive redness that accompany active lesions or remain after acne clears. Also, known as photofacials, IPL uses a broad spectrum of light

FREQUENTLY ASKED QUESTIONS

in the blue and red spectrums, to target melanin (the pigmented cells forming sun spots and pigmentation after acne lesions) and hemoglobin (the red cells that are found in blood vessels and redness that remains after acne lesions). Red and brown marks on the skin can be greatly reduced after a series of IPL treatments. A series of three or four treatments is generally required for the best results. The treatments should be spaced three to five weeks apart to allow proper skin recovery.

62. What is photodynamic therapy?

Photodynamic therapy (PDT) is a special, non-invasive but ablative office treatment for stubborn acne performed with a topical photosensitizing agent called Levulan (5-aminolevulinic or ALA) activated with the blue or red wavelength of light. This is also known as "ALA/PDT treatment". PDT is thought to treat inflamed nodulocystic acne by two separate mechanisms. First, it shrinks the sebaceous (oil-producing) glands of the skin. This reduces acne by decreasing the amount of oil in each pore which feed the infecting bacteria. Photodynamic therapy also directly targets the opportunistic and virulent strain of *P. acnes* bacteria which causes the infection by stimulating the bacteria's protoporphyrin and triggering apoptosis or programmed death of the targeted bacteria. The virulent strain of *P. acnes* bacteria is much higher in metabolic rate than the *P. acnes* strain which is the normal flora, commensal and protective of our skin. This treatment is much more selective in targeting the pathogenic strain of bacteria than topical or systemic antibiotics which kill all bacteria. After PDT treatments, the overall texture of the skin is usually improved. In addition, I find that PDT helps post-inflammatory erythema and hyperpigmentation (the red and brown marks that linger after acne lesions). ALA/PDT treatment also has the unique ability to minimize pores and reduce oil glands, effectively treating stubborn acne vulgaris, acne rosacea, and improve the appearance of some acne scars.

63. When does one suspect an endocrinopathy or hormonal problem in women with acne?

Endocrinopathy should be suspected in a woman with pustular acne eruptions when a female who has never had acne suddenly develops severe acne as a late-onset disorder, or when there is failure to respond to conventional therapy, or when, along with acne, the female shows other signs of hyperandrogenism such as hirsutism, irregular menstruation cycles and changes in voice. A suspicion towards hyperandrogenism is also justified in females with cushinoid features, increased libido, development of acanthosis nigricans, resistance to insulin, progressive weight gain or androgenetic alopecia.

In most women with acne, serum androgens are completely normal. However, it may still be clear that there is a hormonal component to the acne based on history and physical examination. The evidence for this hormonal relationship lies in the fact that their acne flares up prior to menstruation. This relationship is further augmented by the positive response if treated with hormonal therapy. This quandary has led to studies that have found that the levels of serum DHEA-S, testosterone and DHT are higher in women with acne as compared with those without acne. Still, laboratory values may be within the normal range. Minimum tests for endocrine evaluation and interpreting the laboratory values are as follows:

- DHEA-S (adrenal source of androgens):
    » 8000 ng/ml – adrenal tumor;
    » 4000–8000 ng/ml – congenital adrenal hyperplasia.
- Total testosterone (ovarian/adrenal source):
    » 150–200 ng/dl – ovarian tumor;
    » Mild elevations – polycystic ovary disease.
- Luteinizing hormone/follicle-stimulating hormone (LH/FSH):
    » Ratio >2.5 – polycystic ovary disease.

When the source of androgens is the adrenal gland, an elevated level of DHEA-S is observed. An elevation in testosterone commonly indicates that the androgens are of ovarian source. However, one must bear in mind that an elevated testosterone level does not necessarily exclude an adrenal abnormality. In such cases, an additional test, the LH/FSH ratio, can be performed. Establishing identification of an adrenal source of androgens can also be confirmed by an elevated serum level of 17-hydroxyprogesterone, which would be indicative of a congenital adrenal hyperplasia. Furthermore, if the patients were taking oral contraceptives (OCs), it is required that the patients discontinue OC 4–6 weeks prior to endocrine evaluation because OCs would mask any underlying hyperandrogenism. If PCOS is suspected based on presentation, I usually refer the patient to her Gynecologist for an abdominal ultrasound, which is the easiest and least invasive first test.

64. What is Isolaz?

Isolaz is a photopneumatic medical grade technology made by Solta which is used as an in-office procedure that I use very effectively to clear inflamed cystic acne after surgical extraction of inflamed pustules. There are two components to the Isolaz treatment, a variable and adjustable suction that opens the extracted pustules, and an intense pulsed blue or red light, depending on the filter being used, that is delivered to destroy the *P. acnes* bacteria in the extracted pustule and reduce the localized inflammation.

65. Are light-based treatments safe during pregnancy?

There are no studies linking light-based treatments such as LASERs, LED or IPL treatments to birth defects, and practically speaking, such light sources are similar to light from the sun or a light bulb in a lot of ways, so it should not harm the fetus. We often treat patients with surgical extractions and disinfection using blue and red light during pregnancy as-long-as their OB/GYN is also on board and approves the treatment.

66. Can I treat my acne scars while I am still breaking out?

Improving atrophic or hypertrophic acne scarring and post-inflammatory hyperpigmentation require significant trauma to the affected skin to break down, disrupt, promote, remodel dermal collagen and resurface the skin epidermis. Some of the techniques used are various LASERs, subcision, fillers, chemical peels, dermabrasion and microneedling. Trauma required to breakdown existing scarring and remodel and generate new collagen will cause significant inflammation and lead to stimulation of the oil glands and increase in eruptions of new cystic acne lesions which will in turn cause new scarring and hyperpigmentation. I believe that no scarring treatment should be performed until the skin has been cleared of inflammatory acne and has maintained clearance for at least 3 months at which point acne scar treatment can be undertaken with very close attention and care of the skin to help maintain it clear as it recovers from the trauma of the scar treatment to avoid new inflamed eruptions and scarring.

67. What is a chemical peel?

Chemical peeling is a common office procedure that has evolved over the years, using the scientific knowledge of wound healing after controlled chemical skin injury. Chemical peeling is the application of a chemical agent, usually an acid, to the skin. The peeling agent causes a controlled burn and destruction of a part of or the entire epidermis, with or without the dermis, leading to exfoliation and removal of superficial lesions, followed by regeneration of new epidermal and dermal tissues. Indications for chemical peeling include pigmentary disorders, superficial acne scars, aging skin changes, and benign epidermal growths. Contraindications include patients with active bacterial, viral or fungal infection, atrophic skin, abnormal scarring or tendency to keloid formation, facial dermatitis, taking photosensitizing medications, isotretinoin use in the last six months and unrealistic expectations. Since inflamed cystic acne is considered an active bacterial

FREQUENTLY ASKED QUESTIONS

infection, chemical peel as a single modality treatment of such lesions is not effective or a good idea. We include it in our intensive treatment protocol after extraction and disinfection of cysts to stimulate skin turn over and purge the deeper lesions with serial, weekly treatments.

The medium and deep chemical peels should be performed by physician who have completed postgraduate training in dermatology, facial plastic surgery or general plastic surgery. The training for chemical peeling may be acquired during post-graduation or later at a center that provides education and training in cutaneous surgery or in focused workshops providing such training. The physician should have adequate knowledge of the different peeling agents used, the process of wound healing, the technique as well as the identification and management of complications. The physician should provide preoperative counseling and obtain an informed consent in every case with details about the procedure and possible complications and the limitations of the procedure and if more procedures are needed for proper results as well as alternatives.

The depth of penetration and extent of the burn and peeling are determined by several factors including the type, concentration and pH of the acid, proper pre-treatment skin preparation, acid neutralization after treatment, the pressure with which it is applied by the provider, etc. These treatments can be dangerous if not performed correctly by an experienced physician. Superficial peels are considered safe in all skin types. Medium depth peels should be performed with great caution, especially in dark skinned patients. Deep peels are not recommended for dark skin and have a much higher risk of complications and are not appropriate for acne or acne scar treatments. It is essential to do pre-peel priming of the patient's skin with sun protection, use of topical hydroquinone and discontinuation of tretinoin for 2-4 weeks. The physician pays close attention to endpoints in peels to avoid unnecessary complications. A commonly used peel such as Glycolic acid is neutralized after a predetermined duration of time (usually three minutes). However, if erythema or epidermolysis occurs, seen as grayish white appearance of the epidermis or as small blisters, the peel must be immediately neutralized with 10-15% sodium bicarbonate solution, regardless of the duration of application of the peel. The end-point is frosting for TCA peels, which are neutralized either with a neutralizing agent or cold water. For salicylic acid peels, the end-point is the pseudo-frost formed when the salicylic acid crystallizes. Generally, 1-3 coats are applied to get an even frost; it is then washed with water after 3-5 minutes, after the burning has subsided. Jessner solution is applied in 1-3 coats until even frosting is achieved or erythema is seen. Postoperative care includes sun protection and moisturizers. Superficial peels may be repeated weekly or monthly for medium depth peels. In our intensive acne treatment protocol, various superficial and medium depth chemical peels are performed at the end of each session if determined safe to unclog pores and stimulate skin turnover and purging of deeper acne for further extraction and disinfection on weekly basis for the duration of the treatment plan.

68. What is microdermabrasion?

Microdermabrasion is an in-office treatment that removes the outer layer of dead skin cells. The procedure uses a traumatic mechanical abrasion with a burr or crystals in combination with suction. Microdermabrasion causes moderate injury to the skin and is likely to worsen inflammation and lead to increased acne breakout. I do not recommend microdermabrasion on inflamed acne or acne-burdened skin until active acne is cleared as it is likely to cause worsening of inflammatory acne and significant scarring.

69. What is Microneedling?

Microneedling is a minimally invasive cosmetic procedure

that is thought to treat skin concerns via collagen production. Also, known as collagen induction therapy, this treatment may help those looking to reduce the appearance of acne scars and stretch marks. Microneedling instruments vary widely from rollers which work by rolling sharp needles of certain diameter over the skin and creating wedge shaped wounds and pens which insert several needles vertically into the skin at depths ranging from 0.5mm to 3.0mm. The quality and safety of microneedling pens vary widely. No microneedling should be performed on a skin which continues to have inflamed cystic eruptions as the needles which penetrate the pustules will transfer and implant the infection into unaffected adjacent skin and spread the infection. Such treatment will also increase inflammation and exacerbate the eruptions. In my practice, I use a solid-state, microneedling pen with sterile, titanium needle cartridge to breakdown and demolish the firm, rolled edges of atrophic scars in conjunction with subcision and LASER resurfacing to improve the appearance of atrophic acne scars. There is no advantage to improving depressed acne scar by inducing collagen through numerous sessions of microneedling of the dermis across the epidermis when localized collagen loss can be replaced directly and precisely into the dermis with subcision and collagen injection producing immediate improvement.

70. What is Cryotherapy?

Cryotherapy, also called cryosurgery, cryoablation, percutaneous cryotherapy or targeted cryoablation therapy, is a minimally invasive treatment that uses extreme cold to freeze and destroy diseased tissue, ultimately to exfoliate localized areas of skin where the pimples are concentrated. I use this modality in my practice for treatment of inflamed cystic eruptions on chest, back and shoulders where the skin is thicker and better protected from sun exposure after treatment.

Cryotherapy involves the use of liquid nitrogen or carbon dioxide slush to treat acne. The mechanism of destruction in *cryotherapy* is necrosis, which results from the *freezing* and thawing of cells. Treated areas re-epithelialize and heal. Adverse effects of *cryotherapy* are usually minor and short-lived. Typically, liquid nitrogen or solid carbon dioxide is applied to an area of skin, freezing it. Light freezing causes burning and peeling of the skin, moderate freezing causes blistering and hard freezing causes scabbing. This procedure is used as a treatment for acne as well as a method to remove scars and growths and excise some skin cancers. The freezing agent may be sprayed on to the skin or swabbed on, but the end result is the same. Freezing has been found to be a very effective, reliable and relatively inexpensive way to remove most of the surface skin lesions associated with acne. When used as an acne treatment, an area of skin is lightly frozen so, when the top layer of skin is shed, any whiteheads and blackheads that were present are also removed as an effective exfoliant. A cryotherapy treatment may also be used to help pimples heal faster, which has the ultimate effect of reducing any acne scarring. Cryotherapy treatments for acne are usually performed once a week. Side effects of this treatment may include stinging and redness of the skin; there may also be some pain for some period after the treatment. The painful after-effects of cryotherapy may be reduced by applying a steroid to the treated area immediately after the treatment. In very rare cases, a patient with extremely sensitive skin may experience some swelling and blistering after a cryotherapy session. Cryotherapy is also sometimes referred to as cryosurgery and it is, in fact, a form of surgery in the sense that the physician is removing a layer of skin along with the acne blemishes. This method of acne treatment has been available since the 1960s and has proven to be very effective as an acne treatment option but it is not nearly as well known or as widely advertised as over-the-counter medications.

71. Does Hyperbaric Oxygen Therapy (HBOT) have any role in acne treatment?

Hyperbaric means increased atmospheric pressure. At sea level, with the entire earth's atmosphere of air above our heads, we live at an average pressure of 14.7psi (pounds per square inch) or 1 atmosphere. By breathing pure oxygen in a moderately pressurized hyperbaric chamber, dramatically increased amounts of oxygen are safely delivered to all tissues in the body – even to places that have restricted blood flow or blockages. **HBOT** is used in wound healing by improving tissue oxygenation, cellular metabolism, accelerating the healing processes, reducing skin irritations, and producing an anti-inflammatory effect. Oxygen is also able to produces a neo-angiogenisis, or new vessel formation and has an antibacterial effect thanks to its ability to release reactive oxygen species (ROS), compounds that are extremely toxic, as they degrade cellular membranes and cause death of the pathogenic microorganisms. Antibiotics cannot get to the strain of *P. acnes* bacteria that causes pustular acne because it is protected by encapsulation and biofilm. HBOT saturates all of the tissues and fluids of the body with oxygen which shut down the cascade of inflammatory processes triggered by these bacteria, and remove the sources of inflammation that lead to severe and chronic exacerbation of acne breakouts.

Oxygen jump-starts the production of collagen and elastin in the skin. That's why it is likely to speed healing during intensive acne treatment or LASER scar treatment as it regenerates collagen and promotes epithelial cell turnover and recovery. HBOT is especially indicated for sensitive skin that can't tolerate other treatments. Psoriasis and rosacea also respond favorably to oxygen treatments. For severe acne, I recommend clinical oxygen therapy utilizing a pressure of 4 psi (pounds per square inch). This is considered "mild" hyperbaric oxygen therapy, which offers considerable therapeutic benefit to many clients without the potential side effects of treatment at higher pressures. Treatments are performed three times during the first week, twice during the second week and once during the third and subsequent weeks in conjunction with our intensive acne treatments until the acne lesions clear. Milder acne may respond to once-a-week treatment.

72. Which light-based acne treatments are best for teenagers?

PhotoDynamic Therapy and the Isolaz treatment as complements to extraction are both effective and safe for treating acne in teenagers. PDT is not only anti-bacterial, but it is one of the only acne treatments that can decrease sebum production in teenage patients with oily skin. The Isolaz treatment with extraction drains and disinfects pustules and cleans out congested pores. In our experience, these light-based treatments work best in combination with each other and extractions and chemical peels to produce long-lasting improvement. The intensive and structured treatment schedules also reduce the risk of non-compliance in teens, which is a significant contributor to treatment failure for any disease in this population.

73. Is Photodynamic Therapy safe in darker skinned patients?

When performed properly, PDT is safe and effective for treating acne in darker skinned patients. The aminolevulinic acid incubation time (the time the medicine stays on the skin) and the blue LED light treatment time may be adjusted for patients with skin of color. I recommend pre-treating patients with darker skin color with hydroquinone nightly for 3 weeks prior to PDT treatment to avoid hyperpigmentation and be very careful to avoid sun exposure after their PDT treatment to avoid reactivation of aminolevulinic acid and potentially deeper burn.

74. What is a safe treatment for acne during pregnancy?

I generally do not prescribe any oral medications, especially during pregnancy and focus our treatment on the skin and the inflamed, cystic eruptions through hands-on, procedural treatments. The safest treatments during pregnancy are series of light-based treatments such as Isolaz and IPL along with meticulous extraction and disinfection of the cysts while avoiding products that contain tretinoins and use of simple, organic skin care products.

75. Why do depressed acne scars develop?

Acne scars can develop due to release of inflammatory enzymes from pustules and nodulocystic acne which cause disruption and destruction of collagen, leading to atrophy or loss of collagen in the dermis, skin depression and texture deformity. The longer an inflamed lesion sits in the skin, the higher the potential collagen loss. Also, traumatic rupture of pustules with popping or picking will likely lead to more tissue trauma, collagen disruption and scarring.

76. Can my inflamed cystic acne mean that I may have other medical problems?

Acne, one of the most common skin disorders, is also a cardinal component of many systemic diseases or syndromes which should not be missed when initially presenting with acneic eruptions to avoid delay in diagnosis and further morbidity. Acne presents an intriguing model for the study of interactions between hormones, innate immunity, inflammation and wound healing (scarring). The syndromic associations illustrate the nature of these diseases and is suggestive of the pathogenesis of acne. The manifestations and involvement of acne in different systemic diseases and some rare syndromes demonstrate its multifaceted nature. Congenital adrenal hyperplasia (CAH) and seborrhea-acne-hirsutism-androgenetic alopecia (SAHA) syndrome highlight the role of androgenic steroids, while polycystic ovary (PCO) and hyperandrogenism-insulin resistance-acanthosis nigricans (HAIR-AN) syndromes indicate insulin resistance in acne. Apert syndrome with increased fibroblast growth factor receptor 2 (FGFR2) signaling results in follicular hyperkeratinization and sebaceous gland hypertrophy in acne. Synovitis-acne-pustulosis-hyperostosis-osteitis (SAPHO) and pyogenic arthritis-pyoderma gangrenosum-acne (PAPA) syndromes highlight the attributes of inflammation to acne formation. A serious approach to every individual's acneic eruptions requires a commitment to observation, review of history and proper diagnosis and treatment planning by a physician specializing in the treatment of acne.

77. How can I remove the red marks left behind after adult acne?

Post-inflammatory erythema, or the red marks left behind after acne are usually reactive and resolve spontaneously once the source of inflammation is treated. We tell our patients that it is like smoke during a fire and as the fire is put out, the smoke usually clears. If persistent, it can be treated with IPL in the red-light spectrum, KTP or V-Beam laser. Two or three treatments may usually be sufficient for greatly reducing the post-inflammatory erythema.

78. What causes "post-inflammatory hyperpigmentation"?

Post-Inflammatory Hyperpigmentation (PIH) results from an increase of skin pigment, melanin, production after skin stress caused by infection or injury, especially from sun damage. In layman's terms, PIH is when the skin becomes discolored or darkened in an area that was recently inflamed, like a painful acne cyst. Inflammatory acne lesions can cause post-inflammatory hyperpigmentation, particularly in skin of color. We tell our patients that it is like the ashes after a fire. The fire was the breakout (inflammatory acne) and the ashes are remnants of the fire (PIH) that indicate where the pimples used to be. These remnants can sometimes stick around for many months without treatment. The best way to treat them is to prevent them by treating inflamed cystic eruptions immediately and intensively. PIH generally resolves spontaneously in 3-4 months if no further inflammation and with strict sun protection.

FREQUENTLY ASKED QUESTIONS

79. How long does PIH stay after acne has resolved?

Post-inflammatory Hyperpigmentation (PIH) can improve with time, but without treatment it may linger for 6-12 months or longer. Topical prescription medications, such as hydroquinone, Kojic acid and tazarotene can be used to improve the appearance of PIH. Chemical peels such as Jessner formulations and laser treatment, such as Fractional CO_2 laser and especially 1927nm fractionated thulium laser by Fraxel are very effective in treating PIH.

80. Does my acne need to be completely clear prior to having laser treatment for acne scars?

Acne scars may be treated once the acne is cleared to avoid exacerbation of the inflammation causing new breakouts and further scarring. Although many individuals may be focused on their scars, the most important factor is the health of the skin. A clear and healthy skin is the foundation upon which all attempts at improving appearance should be based. It is my experience that acne scar treatments are likely to fail if performed on a skin that continues to be distressed and challenged with chronic inflammation.

81. Should I take dietary supplements or vitamins to help clear my acne?

Vitamin are co-enzymes which allow enzymes to function optimally when breaking down proteins and carbohydrates. Unless an individual has significant intestinal malabsorption or a very poor diet, Vitamins and antioxidant pills don't work, and at best are ineffective and at worst, may be harmful and highly toxic. In fact, self-treating with vitamins is more likely harming rather than helping your body. In 1954, Rebeca Gerschman, first identified vitamins as a possible danger – ideas expanded upon by Denham Harman, from the Donner Laboratory of Medical Physics at UC Berkeley in 1956, who argued that free radicals can lead to cellular deterioration, disease and, ultimately, ageing. The process starts with mitochondria, those tiny combustion engines that sit within our cells. Inside their internal membranes food and oxygen are converted into water, carbon dioxide, and energy. This is respiration, a mechanism that fuels all complex life.

In the 1970s and into the 80s, many laboratory experiments on mice demonstrated that an excess of antioxidants didn't quell the ravages of ageing, nor stop the onset of disease. Subsequently, long-term double-blind controlled clinical trials were conducted in humans trying to figure out what antioxidant supplementation does for our health and survival. The results are far from heartening where incidence of lung, breast and prostate cancers increased in those taking the supplements compared to placebo. Current findings provide ample grounds to discourage use of medically unnecessary supplemental in those with access to healthy diet. Antioxidants have a dark side. There is increasing evidence that free radicals themselves are essential for our health. We now know that free radicals are often used as molecular messengers that send signals from one region of the cell to another. In this role, they have been shown to modulate when a cell grows, when it divides in two, and when it dies. At every stage of a cell's life, free radicals are vital. Without them, cells would continue to grow and divide uncontrollably. There's a word for this; cancer. We would also be more prone to infections from outside. When under stress from an unwanted bacterium or virus, free radicals are naturally produced in higher numbers, acting as silent alarms for our immune system. In response, those cells at the vanguard of our immune defense – macrophages and lymphocytes – start to divide and scout out the problem. If it is a bacterium, they will engulf and trap it, but it is not yet dead. To change that, free radicals are once again called into action. Inside the immune cell, they are used for what they are infamous for, to damage and to kill. The intruder is torn apart. Therefore, a healthy immune response depends on free radicals and removing them with antioxidants would theoretically, leave the body helpless against some infections. The body normally filters excess free radicals out of the bloodstream into urine for disposal. Our bodies have been selected to balance the risk of oxygen ever since the first microbes started to breathe this toxic gas. We can't change billions of years of evolution with a simple pill. No one would deny that vitamin C is vital to a healthy lifestyle, as are all antioxidants, but unless you are following doctor's orders, these supplements are rarely going to be the answer for a longer life or treatment of an infection such as acne when a healthy diet is a much better option. Administration of antioxidants is justified only when it is evident that there is a real deficiency of a specific vitamin or antioxidant. The best option is to get antioxidants from food because it contains a mixture of antioxidants that work best together.

Vitamins can interfere with absorption and function of other medications as well as lead to tissue injury directly. Too much vitamin A (in its retinol form) may lead to liver failure or even death, while pregnant women may risk birth defects. Overdoing vitamin D intake may lead to unhealthy weight loss, bone pain, vomiting, diarrhea and muscle problems. Vitamin E overdose may increase a person's risk of bleeding, especially for those taking blood-thinning medication. Too much vitamin K may harm people with kidney or liver disease. An iron overdose from supplements could damage organ function, leading to death if untreated. Additionally, significant Lead, mercury and arsenic contaminants have been detected in vitamins and dietary supplements imported into U.S. as the manufacturers have no regulations or oversight in their own countries and the USFDA does not regulate vitamins and dietary supplements. Over time and in large doses, such heavy metal contaminants may be toxic especially in young individuals.

82. Do heat and humidity cause acne breakouts?

Heat and humidity increase skin inflammation and stimulate more sebum production which can lead to comedonal oil gland congestion as well as worsening of inflamed cystic acne. We generally advise that our patients avoid heat or steam to the acne-burdened skin and to use cold compress to reduce inflammation.

83. Does smoking cause acne or make it worse?

There's not yet a definitive answer to this question. It seems for every study that claims smoking can result in an acne breakout, there's another study that disproves this theory. The medical research community requires a great deal more research before any true consensus can be drawn. While the debate rages on about whether or not smoking causes, or aggravates the prevalence of acne blemishes, the science is clear about smoking's negative effects on the skin and health in general. Regular smoking constricts the blood vessels, disrupt our hormone balance, damages the immune system, slows down the healing of wounds and damages the surface of many parts of our bodies. From psoriasis to aging, skin cancer to your skin's ability to heal, smoking can wreak havoc on the skin. Conflicting evidence about cigarettes and acne vulgaris aside, there is one form of acne that does have a known relationship with smoking: acne inversa.

84. What is Acne Inversa?

Acne Inversa, also known as Hidradenitis supuritiva or ingrown hair, is a chronic skin condition involving the infection and inflammation of the apocrine sweat glands, forming pustular bumps often mistaken for acne; whereas, acne vulgaris is due to infection and inflammation of the sebaceous or oil gland. Acne inversa tend to recur in specific regions of the body such as intertriginous skin, which refers to areas in which two separate patches of skin touch such as in the underarms, between buttocks cheeks, under the foreskin, and in the vagina and can be very painful and often leave behind deep scar tissue when they heal.

FREQUENTLY ASKED QUESTIONS

85. Will touching my face cause acne?

Touching your face can trigger breakouts because some breakouts are triggered by bacteria, and our hands are breeding ground for bacteria Our hands are consistently touching all things that are not necessarily clean. If you're touching existing breakouts and then touching other parts of your face, you can spread bacteria if the acne is at a pustule stage. Our hands are also constantly touching many animals and objects which are contaminated with various microorganisms, some of which can cause infections. When touching our face frequently, we can transfer these organisms from other animals and objects or even from other areas of our own body where pustules have erupted. It is also advised to clean hands before inserting a finger into a jar of a product which will then be applied to our skin as the organisms may transfer to the product which will be a reservoir of the spread of infection upon reapplication. We advise individuals with acne-burdened skin to clean or replace their makeup brushes frequently and disinfect their shaver after every use to prevent recontamination of face and possible exacerbation or spread of infection, cleaning of hands or surfaces which come into contact with skin using water and avoid repeated use of strong sanitizers and disinfectants as they are not necessary and may cause skin irritation. It is also advised to avoid skin care products that are in open jars as they are more likely to become contaminated with repeated use.

86. Are sunscreens safe for acne-burdened individuals with inflamed cystic eruptions?

Contrary to what we are told by many doctors, there is a growing body of evidence in the literature that suggests sunscreens contain many toxic and teratogenic (birth defect) and potentially carcinogenic (cancer) chemicals which may be highly dangerous to the compromised, acne-burdened skin especially with repeated and prolonged exposure. Inflammatory cystic acne eruptions cause the skin to become brittle or fragile with increased sensitivity due to disruption of the protective keratin barrier. No sunscreens are safe as only sun avoidance and physical barriers such as large hats, sunbrellas and SPF-rated, engineered clothing are safe for protecting the acne-burdened skin against the sun's oxidative damage. The less we depend on chemicals for environmental protection, the healthier our skin and our body will be to combat and recover from disease.

While the idea of FDA-approved sunscreens being harmful is a highly controversial topic, the current world literature is replete with reports of absorption and toxicity of various chemicals in sunscreen formulations. Natural sunscreens contain physical or mineral protectants such as *zinc* and *titanium dioxide*. Mineral sunscreens, mainly made up of titanium dioxide and zinc oxide, sit on the top of the skin and physically deflect damaging UV rays away from the skin but become highly toxic and irritating if absorbed into the skin and blood through open wounds such as acne eruptions; whereas, chemical sunscreens work by absorbing UV rays, converting them into heat, and then releasing it, presenting potential concerns of toxicity and photostability and break down in the presence of UV and generation of free radicals. These products work by being applied generously and frequently, which increase toxic exposure and systemic absorption risk. Chemical sunscreens contain ingredients such as Octinoxate, oxybenzone, avobenzone, octocrylene, octisalate, homosalate, benzophenone, and methyl anthranilate which are a few of the highly questionable petrochemicals, can be harmful to the environment and can be endocrine disruptors when applied in large amounts.

Sunscreens are designed to include ingredients to enhance skin adherence and penetration, resulting in measurable absorption of sunscreen chemicals in blood, breast milk, and urine. In addition to absorption through the skin, these chemicals can potentially be inhaled when sprayed. Added fragrances such as Phthalates and other mystery ingredients and fixatives commonly found in fragrances are unstable and tend to oxidize, break down

FREQUENTLY ASKED QUESTIONS

and have been linked to reproductive disorders, endocrine disruption, and allergies.

Considering that tens of thousands of tons of sunscreen lotions are washed into the oceans, the chemicals in even one drop of sunscreen are enough to damage fragile coral reef systems. The most damaging of the chemicals is oxybenzone which not only kills most of the coral, but causes DNA damage in adults and deforms the DNA in coral in the larval stage, making it unlikely they can develop properly. When zinc oxide and titanium dioxide nanoparticles wash off skin, they enter the environment, with unknown effects. The implications of nanoparticle pollution for the environment have not been sufficiently assessed. The potential negative environmental effects of nanoscale and conventional zinc and titanium should be carefully studied and weighed against the environmental impact of other UV blockers. Sunscreen ingredients have been shown to damage coral, accumulate in fish and the environment, and disrupt hormones in fish and amphibians.

Although previous research has concluded that metal oxide nanoparticles do not penetrate healthy skin, it remains contentious whether this conclusion holds under normal conditions of sunscreen use as recent studies have demonstrated toxic blood levels of zinc and titanium oxide, especially as a nanoparticle formulation smaller than 30 microns in size. Metal oxide absorption pose numerous risks including neurotoxicity and repeated application of such compounds to an acne-burdened skin with significantly compromised keratin barrier will likely result in dangerous levels of skin and blood stream absorption of such metal oxides. Such metal oxides **can also cause lung damage including cancer when inhaled.** The lungs have difficulty clearing small particles, so the particles may pass from the lungs into the bloodstream. Insoluble nanoparticles that penetrate skin or lung tissue can cause extensive organ damage, which is of relevance to acne-burdened skin.

CHAPTER **12**

Tips & Pearls

1. Inflamed cystic acne is not genetic. There is no "acne gene" identified and although many inherited conditions may contribute to the severity of an individual's inflammatory response, pustular acne is an infection of the oil glands caused by a virulent and opportunistic strain of *P. acnes* which is different from the strain that forms our skin's protective microbiome. Acne is a disease, not a curse and can be cleared when treated by a physician specializing in the treatment of acne. Clear and healthy skin is your birth right, not inflamed, pustular acne.

2. Visit your acne specialist doctor as soon as acne develops. Delaying treatment for even mild acne can lead to scarring and discoloration.

3. Don't pop pimples at home – this can cause more inflammation and scarring of the skin.

4. LASER and light treatments are great for teenagers who are often non-compliant with home-care.

5. Wear loose cotton clothing while working out, to help prevent body acne. Backpack straps, Helmets and chin straps can cause

repeated skin trauma and irritation as well as serving as a reservoir of bacteria which can cause skin infection.

6. Washing skin with a salicylic acid cleanser after working out can help to control body acne and inflammation.

7. Washing with Soaps containing Salicylic acid and sulfur help control acne on torso.

8. Occasional 20-minute bleach bath soak helps disinfect the torso and limbs of bacterial contamination.

9. It's better for both members of an intimate couple to treat their acne together to avoid recirculation or recontamination with the bacteria causing acne.

10. You can only maintain clear if you start from clear.

11. Avoid creamy make up and use powder formulations.

12. Avoid sunscreen lotion or spray while breaking out or undergoing intensive acne treatment.

13. Minimize or avoid use of benzoyl peroxide.

14. Avoid heat and steam when experiencing inflamed pustular eruptions.

15. A low glycemic index diet may help to reduce acne inflammation. Cut back on processed foods and add leafier green vegetables and berries to your diet.

16. Avoid medically unnecessary vitamins and dietary supplements which at best, have no positive impact on acne and at worst and most likely may be dangerous to your health.

17. Don't start making major diet changes to clear acne unless your diet is objectively unhealthy or you have gastrointestinal stress caused by specific foods causing increased inflammation.

18. Don't start intensive acne scar treatments until acne is cleared and maintaining clear.

19. Avoid experimenting on your skin with various acne and skin care products.

20. Avoid suppressive, chemical treatments such as prolonged oral antibiotics or birth control pills to manage your acne.

21. For sun protection, I recommend physical protection using, large hats, umbrellas and spf-rated clothing instead of chemical sunscreen.

22. If you have a pimple and need it gone fast, see your acne specialist doctor for a cortisone injection, which can flatten your pimple in 24-48 hours. Keep in mind that depression and loss of pigmentation may occur at the site of injection.

23. Apply ice to reduce pain and swelling of an inflamed pustule. As soon as you notice the cyst, wrap an ice cube in a paper towel and apply it to the area for 5 to 10 minutes. Repeat this two more times, with 10-minute breaks between icing. Apply a warm compress once the pustules comes to a head. To make a warm compress, soak a clean washcloth in hot water; make sure the water isn't too hot to avoid burning your skin. Then, apply the warm compress to the pimple for 10 to 15 minutes. Do this three to four times daily until the pimple releases pus and heals.

24. If it doesn't seem like acne, it might be something else such as Rosacea or Pityrosporum folliculitis. Consult a physician

specializing in diagnosis and treatment of acne to avoid misdiagnosis and delay in treatment.

25. Blue and red light therapy are safe and effective acne treatment options during pregnancy.

26. Unlike retinoids and salicylic acid, glycolic and lactic acid cleansers can safely be used during pregnancy.

27. Acne-like bumps on the beard are not always acne. It may be a condition called pseudofolliculitis barbae.

28. Consult an experienced doctor if you are not sure.

29. Products are best used for keeping skin clear as they are not often effective in clearing acne.

30. Look at your skin care products and if they contain fragrance it may be time to look for a different brand. Synthetic fragrances contain many ingredients that may be irritating to your skin.

31. Remain diligent and compliant with the intensive acne treatment schedule for best outcome.

32. "moisturizers" help reduce loss of internal skin moisture and thus act as "anti-desiccants" and not really as moisturizers that push moisture into the dermis.

33. Apply moisturizer while the skin is still moist after washing.

34. Avoid sun exposure for 48 hours after Photodynamic Therapy to avoid deeper burn.

35. Use an organic, foaming cleanser that doesn't need to be rubbed

or scrubbed into the skin to lather. Rubbing and scrubbing the skin can cause further irritation and inflammation.

36. Don't "pop" or rupture your pustules to avoid scarring or worsening of infection. If you are not able to book an appointment promptly with your acne doctor, you may apply ice to the pustule for several minutes, and carefully extract the cyst content by making a small opening using a clean lancet, then gently scrub clean with Hibiclense to disinfect the pustule followed by application of moisturizer to protect the wound.

37. Stay away from spa facials where the esthetician extracts pustules by "popping" them with fingers and massages oils and heavy creams into your face.

38. Inflamed cystic acne is a disease requiring intensive medical treatment and not a cosmetic condition to be treated by a cosmetologist or esthetician.

39. If you tend to pick and squeeze your pimples, avoid looking into mirrors during the day.

40. Wash and clean makeup brushes often to clear them of bacteria and debris that can lead to bacterial skin contamination.

41. Do not shave the acne-burdened skin with sharp razor to avoid skin irritation. Use electric shavers and then wash the blades under running warm to hot water or alcohol before putting it away.

42. Make sure to wash your hands before applying your makeup or skin care products. The oils and bacteria on your fingers may be contributing to your acne breakouts.

43. Don't sleep in your makeup. If you're too tired to wash your face, use a makeup remover pad.

44. Use magnified mirrors only to double-check complete removal of make-up.

45. Do not use products that come in jars and instead use products provided in tubes or pumps to minimize the risk of bacterial contamination.

46. Beware of "Noncomedogenic" Claims. Noncomedogenic is a fancy way of saying a product won't clog your pores. There is no official FDA definition of the term noncomedogenic or a defined list of ingredients proven not to clog pores as Dr. Fulton's claims based on rabbit ear model experiments have been largely discredited. The best bet is to look for oil-free products that don't contain additional ingredients like artificial fragrances and preservatives, as these commonly cause skin reactions.

47. Wipe your cell phone down daily with an alcohol swab to kill any bacteria and reduce oils that may get transferred onto your skin.

48. To avoid skin picking, apply cold compress to the skin to reduce inflammation and discomfort.

49. Wash your hands before washing your face.

50. Strongly consider Photodynamic Therapy or our Intensive hands-on acne treatment if you have inflamed cystic acne.

51. Avoid Do-it-yourself acne treatments that can make your skin worse.

52. Exfoliate without scrubbing. Use gentle enzymes or fruit acid

wipes to exfoliate and keep pores open without traumatizing the skin with scrubbing which increases skin inflammation and oil production. I generally recommend a grapefruit extract wipe, 2-3 times weekly before bed to maintain a healthy skin turnover and minimize pore clogging.

53. Don't do microdermabrasion or microneedling if you are still breaking out as they will likely worsen the infection.

54. Rosacea patients can often benefit from sulfur-based washes and IPL treatments.

55. Keep a diary of past medications so you will be able to look up what worked and what didn't in case you choose to undergo intensive acne treatment.

56. Use foundation with Salicylic Acid, such as Oxygenetix, to keep pores open.

57. Don't stop your acne treatment series prematurely just because you achieve clear.

58. Hormonal pattern acne is best treated with intensive hands-on procedures and Spironolactone. Avoid systemic hormonal birth control.

59. LASERs are a useful tool in improving skin texture irregularity due to atrophic scars, not in treating inflamed cystic acne.

60. Do not wait to "outgrow" acne, seek treatment now.

61. One size does not fit all for acne treatment. Make sure you have a customized, intensive regimen which adjusts to your acne's changing condition and your skin's changing needs.

62. Check out your acne written and photo diary to track your progress.

63. Avoid alcohol if you are taking oral antibiotics or experiencing dry skin.

64. Over consumption of caffeine may cause skin dehydration and hormonal stimulation which may worsen acne.

65. Do not use tobacco in any shape or form.

66. If you are overweight, try to get back to your ideal weight. Obesity is associated with worsening acne.

67. Seeking intensive treatment for acne early can decrease the chance of having scars later.

68. Redness associated with inflamed cystic acne will improve spontaneously when the acne is cleared.

69. Both green tea and tea tree oils are good natural ingredients that may help fight acne infection.

70. Chemical peels will stimulate skin turn over and further breakout.

71. Organic Witch Hazel astringent and Apple Cider Vinegar are excellent, non-irritating skin cleansers.

72. Don't share your acne medications with anyone and do not self-treat your acne with a friend's products, left-over or expired antibiotics.

73. If you pick your skin and it starts bleeding, scrub with Hibiclense and put antibiotic ointment on the wound to prevent cellulitis and scab from forming.

74. Patients with chronic psuedofolliculitis barbae (Razor bumps), may consider Photodynamic Therapy before undergoing permanent laser hair removal if they wish to maintain the option of growing facial hair in the future.

75. Acne can occur on the buttock, and legs, and those areas often do well with bleach bath, sulfur soap and benzoyl peroxide wash.

76. Photodynamic Therapy can also be used to clear back and body acne.

77. There are several acne imposters such as rosacea and pityrosporum folliculitis. If your acne is not responding to traditional therapy or is new in onset, be sure that your doctor considers another diagnosis.

78. New onset hormonal-pattern, adult cystic acne should be investigated by a doctor for endocrine disorders.

79. Food allergies and sensitivities, enzyme deficiencies and Small Intestinal Bacterial Overgrowth (SIBO) should be investigated in any Acne sufferer with history of Gastrointestinal distress.

80. Only registered dieticians and physicians are qualified to provide dietary advice.

81. For patients who are prone to ingrown hairs, try shaving after showering and using special skin brushes to free the hair follicle from under the skin. The steam will help soften the skin and make razor bumps less likely.

82. Patients with keratosis pilaris (bumps on upper arms) will often benefit by using a peel pad that contains salicylic and glycolic acid and moisturize daily.

83. Don't wash your skin too aggressively or use m
    or harsh scrubs. Remember it is not dirt that caus
    much washing can lead to irritation and increase i

84. Always bring a list of your past medications (bo
    and non-prescription) to your first appointment w   the doctor
    specializing in acne treatment.

85. Knowledge is power. The more you know about acne and its treatments, the better chance of success you will have. If the treatment doesn't make sense, then don't do it.

86. You don't have to pollute your body with dangerous chemicals to clear your skin.

CHAPTER **13**

Glossary of Terms & Definitions

Acne
Also, known as acne vulgaris is a common skin condition made up of one or more lesions scattered on the face, back, buttocks, or anywhere on the body where sebaceous glands and hair follicles exist. Acne can appear in many different forms including: open comedones (blackheads), closed comedones (whiteheads), papules (red bumps), pustules (pus bumps), and cysts (painful deep nodules).

Acne cosmetica
The medical term that describes a condition in which acne is caused or worsened by use of specific skincare and makeup products.

Acne detergicans
Acne that is caused or flared by hyperkeratosis resulting from over-use of certain types of skin cleansers or by using too strong of a cleanser for the skin type.

Acne excoriée
A complicated condition of acne that is caused by the client constantly picking and scraping at the skin, often with the fingernails. It Is characterized by round, flat lesions that are often hyperpigmented or red.

Acne mechanica
Acne that is worsened or flared due to physical pressure and friction on the skin.

GLOSSARY OF TERMS & DEFINITIONS

Acne scars
Residual damage to the skin results from inflammatory acne vulgaris. Acne scars can be hypertrophic (i.e. raised) or atrophic (i.e. depressed) which are often described as "ice pick", "box car" or "rolling", these scars are permanent and can only be changed by physical treatment. When the body has a vigorous response, almost inappropriately strong, to acne bacteria, this can lead to inflammation. Intense inflammation over time can cause collagen disruption and destruction leading to scarring. Some people are more prone to scarring than others. Some patients with intense inflammation can end up with significant, deforming scars.

Acne Venenata or Contact Acne
Acne that is related to exposure to certain substances.

Adapalene
Synthetically produced retinoid, considered to be the least irritating of the topical retinoids for acne.

Adrenal androgens
Male hormones produced in the adrenal cortex. These include testosterone and DHEA.

Adrenal glands
Sit on top of the kidneys and produce several types of hormones including adrenaline and noradrenalin, two important hormones that regulate nerve transmission and the heart rate. Adrenaline and noradrenalin are both also secreted when the body is under extreme stress, such as an emergency.

Adrenocorticotrophic hormone (ACTH)
Hormones secreted by the pituitary gland. which stimulates the adrenal gland to produce androgens,

Aldosterone
Which helps the kidney reabsorb water and sodium during the blood filtering process.

Alipidic
Means lack of lipids and refers to skin that does not produce enough sebum.

Allergies
The rejection of a specific substance by the body's immune system.

5-alpha reductase
An enzyme produced by the skin and reproductive organs that will convert testosterone to an even more powerful form of male hormone.

Anaerobic
Describes bacteria that cannot survive in the presence of oxygen.

Androgens
Male sex / reproductive hormones.

Astringent
Also known as toner, used to remove excess oil and dirt from the skin.

Atrophic Scars
Scars that appear as depressions in the skin. Formed as a result of thinning or loss of subdermal tissue such as collagen creating a depressed or pitted mark left behind after acne. Examples include "Rolling", "Box Car" or "ice pick" scarring.

Barrier function
The protection function against dehydration and penetration of irritants through the skin due to the presence of the lipid matrix between epidermal cells.

Basal layer
The only live layer of the epidermis located at the base of the epidermis just above the papillary dermis.

Basement membrane
Another term for the papillary dermis.

Benzoyl Peroxide
A bleach and a common ingredient in many acne-fighting topical products that works as an antimicrobial to help kill *P. acnes* anaerobic

bacteria by releasing oxygen used to improve acne lesions such as papules and pustules sometimes in combination with other products such as antibiotics in prescription formulations.

Blackhead
Open comedone with no inflammation. Can be raised or flat on the skin with a dark center. Contains clogged pore filled with sebum, dead cells and sometimes bacteria. The surface is black because the contents inside become oxidized from the outside air.

Blue Light Therapy
Blue light is a physical acne treatment that works by directly killing Propionibacterium acnes (*P. acnes*), the acne causing bacteria. Blue light is often administered through LED lights. It can be performed in doctor's office.

Carbohydrates
Break down to basic chemical sugars which are the sole source of nutritional energy for the body.

Cell renewal or keratinization process
The 28-day cycle in which cells migrate from the basal cell layer to the corneum.

Chemical exfoliation
Use of chemicals (often acids) to remove dead cell buildup from the skin surface.

Chemical Peels
A treatment performed in a doctor's office that is aimed to treat fine lines, pigment (brown spots), photo-damage, melasma, active acne and sometimes acne scars. The process involves causing a localized and controlled burn by applying a chemical agent to the skin for a specified amount of time in order to remove the epidermis (top layer of skin) and stimulate collagen remodeling.

Chloracne
A relatively rare type of severe acne caused by exposure to chemical derivatives of chlorine known as chlorinated hydrocarbons.

Cleansing milks
Non-foaming cleansers primarily used for makeup removal.

Closed comedones
Also known as whiteheads, appear as small bumps just under the skin surface. Closed comedones have very small follicle opening and contain plugs of dead cells and solidified sebum.

Collagen
Protein structure prevalent in the skin responsible for skin firmness.

Comedone
Mixture of dead cells (corneocytes) and solidified sebum forms a plug in a sebaceous follicle. (plural: comedones).

Comedogenic
Products or ingredients that are known to cause hyperkeratosis in the follicle leading to the development of comedones. When an individual develops comedones due to use of a skin care product, this is known as a comedogenic reaction.

Comedogenicity
The tendency of certain topical substances to trigger hyperkeratosis and the development of comedones.

Comedolytic
Refers to treatments or substances that can loosen or break loose or prevent comedones.

Comedonal acne
Involves the development of whitehead and blackhead lesions resulting from follicle impactions. These are non-inflammatory and different from pustules and Nodulocystic acne which are inflammatory and are caused by bacterial infection of the oil glands.

Corneocytes
keratin-filled cells within the stratum corneum.

Cortisone injections
A brief in-office treatment performed to quickly reduce the appearance

of active acne. A medication called triamcinolone is injected at a low concentration directly into an inflammatory papule or cyst (aka "pimple"). This procedure takes only a minute and is relatively pain-free. Over the next 24 hours, the pimple will improve significantly and flatten out. This is the most effective spot treatment for acutely inflamed acne.

Cosmetic
As defined by the FDA, is "an article intended to be rubbed, poured, sprinkled, or otherwise applied to the human body or any part thereof for cleansing, beautifying, promoting attractiveness, or altering the appearance."

Cyst
A boil-like lesion which consists of a sac lined with epithelium or skin cells below the skin in the dermis, that is filled with white blood cells, bacteria and/or pus.

Dead skin cells
Layers of the epidermis that are constantly renewing. The top, superficial layer sheds and the bottom layers of the epidermis rise to the top to continue the cycle. Dead skin cells sometimes stick inside the pores, forming plugs that can lead to acne.

De-fatting
A procedure used before many peels that uses solvents such as acetone to remove any surface sebum or oily debris that can interfere with uniform penetration of a chemical peeling agent.

Dehydrated
Refers to a condition in which the skin is not holding enough moisture, which can result in flaking, rough textures and accentuated wrinkles.

Demodex folliculorum
A type of skin mite that is often present in cases of rosacea.

Dendrites
Tentacle like cellular branches.

Dendritic cells
antigen-presenting **cells** of the immune system which process antigen material and present it to the T **cells** of the immune system to identify and mount an immune response.

Deoxyribonucleic acid
Better known as DNA the "blueprint" material that contain all the information that run the function of every living cell.

Dermis
The deeper layer of skin, located under the epidermis (top layer of skin) and above the subcutaneous layer, where hair follicles, sebaceous glands and fibroblasts are located. Gives strength and elasticity to the skin.

Desmosomes
Tiny attachments between cells.

Desquamation
The process in which the corneum sheds continuously.

Desincrustant
Specialized product that causes softening of the fatty follicular plug.

Desincrustation
A procedure that softens the hardened sebaceous deposits in comedones or sebaceous filaments.

Desquamate
The process of dead skin cells releasing from the skin surface.

Differentiation
The process in which basal cells develop into other types of epidermal cells.

Dihydrotestosterone (DHT)
Potent form of testosterone. responsible for skin oiliness.

Disaccharide
Carbohydrate made up of two molecular sugar units.

Drug
As defined by the FDA, is an article (ingredient) "intended to affect the structure or any function of the body."

Drug facts label
A standardized label required to be on all OTC drugs that clearly states the active ingredients, directions, precautions for use, warnings, and a list of the Inactive ingredients.

Elastin
Protein structure that helps the skin stretch and "snap back" to its normal state.

Elastosis
Lack of elasticity resulting in skin sagging.

Endocrine glands
The body's system of glands that produce hormones that regulate and affect many body functions from growth and metabolism to sexual function.

Endometrium
The lining of the uterus that is formed during the menstrual cycle, and broken down during menstruation.

Environmental factors
Outside of genetic and hormonal factors, that can cause or negatively affect acne conditions or contribute to complications in clearing the skin.

Epidermis
The outermost, top layer of the skin, supported by the underlying dermis. The outermost layer of the epidermis is made up of dead skin cells, which rise to the top and flake off.

Epodermolysis
Medical term for a blister.

Epigaltocatechin-3-gallate (EGCG)
A phytochemical in green tea which is a strong antioxidant and

anti-inflammatory botanical chemical that reduces inflammation and may offer properties that indirectly regulate levels of hormonal dihydrotestosterone, which is a sebum-stimulant and acne trigger.

Erythematotelangiectatic rosacea
Characterized by red patchy areas in the cheeks, and frequent redness and blushing, often referred to as 'dry rosacea."

Essential amino acids
Building blocks of proteins and amino acids that must be part of the diet, as the body cannot manufacture these.

Estrogen or estradiol
The best-known female hormone, produced by the ovaries.

Excoriating
Self-picking at acne lesions causing skin damage.

Exfoliation
The process of removing dead skin cells chemically (such as chemical peels or peel pads) or physically (such as microscrubs or microdermabrasion).

Extractions
A method that manually removes sebum, dead cells, pus and bacteria from within pustules or comedones. Often performed using a comedone extractor or a small needle / lancet to open the cyst and then a loop to gently push the cyst contents or comedone impaction out through the small opening.

Fats
Also, known as lipids, can be used by the body as energy. lipids are used by the body to make hormones, to create cell membranes, and are important for absorption of fat-soluble vitamins A, D, E, and K.

Favre-Racouchot syndrome
A disease that presents with a constellation of large open and closed comedones, primarily around the eye area, upper cheeks, and sometimes the forehead. This type of acne is formally associated with very severe sun damage.

Fiber
A carbohydrate, which is necessary for proper digestion. Fiber is made of a carbohydrate called cellulose, which is not digested by humans, and is important in helping push wastes out of the colon.

Fibroblasts
Specialized cells in the reticular dermis that produce both collagen and elastin fibrils.

Fitzpatrick Skin Typing
A universal scale to classify the level of pigment in the skin. This typing also determines a person's resistance to sun burn and sun damage as well as predicting response to chemical peels or LASERs.

Flares of rosacea
Refers to episodes when the symptoms of rosacea are pronounced.

Fordyce spots
Whitish-yellow bumps that can occur on the edge of your lips or inside your cheeks, also called Fordyce granules or Fordyce glands, are enlarged oil glands. They are completely normal, harmless, and painless. Infection of these glands can present as inflamed cystic acne eruptions.

Fractional CO_2
A safe and effective treatment for skin resurfacing to improve superficial scars and wrinkles. This wavelength of this laser pokes tiny microscopic holes in the skin and is mainly absorbed by the water in the dermis. These holes cause new collagen to be generated, which tighten and smoothen skin.

Fraxel
A line of ablative and non-ablative LASERs for skin resurfacing and rejuvenation developed by Solta Medical in 2000. Fraxel LASERs cause fractional photothermolysis of skin (leaving normal skin in between treated areas to speed up healing) used to treat a range of skin conditions such as fine lines, wrinkles, sun damage, acne scars, and dark pigmentation including melasma. Different Fraxel systems use

different wavelengths such as: 10,600 nm CO2 (Re:pair), 1550 nm Erbium, and 1927 nm Thulium lasers (Dual).

Fulguration
Frequently called sparking, is the application of high frequency to individual acne lesions.

Galvanic desincrustation
The use of a very mild galvanic current to penetrate the desincrustant product deeper into the follicle.

Glucocorticoids
Steroids, commonly known as cortisone or cortisol, and are best known for responding to stress. Cortisol is produced to deal with stress, increases blood sugar levels, and affects both protein and lipid levels in the bloodstream.

Glucose
A type of sugar and basic unit of a carbohydrate.

Glycemic index
A measure of the release time of blood sugar for a specific food.

Glycosaminoglycans
Polysaccharide carbohydrate chains that make up the ground substance.

Ground substance
A jelly-like fluid that fills the spaces between elastin and collagen fibrils. Along with fat, also helps surround and protect blood vessels, lymph vessels and nerves present in the reticular layer.

Hair Follicles
Small channel where hair grows. Opens up to the surface of a pore. Can be blocked by multiple hairs, bacteria or pus.

High-glycemic foods
Foods that cause release of an abundance of blood sugar in a short period of time

High frequency
An electrical treatment that improves skin circulation and creates a tiny amount of surface ozone that can kill bacteria.

Hormone Replacement Therapy (HRT)
Oral birth control, sometimes used to raise estrogen levels to reduce sebum production for acne management or other unwanted symptoms of perimenopause.

Hyaluronic Acid
A strong hydrating molecule that holds up to 1,000 times its own weight in water, is one of these polysaccharides.

Hyperpigmentation
Overproduction of melanin that causes dark spots or splotches to form on the skin surface.

Hypertrophic Scars
A type of acne scar more common on back and chest. These scars are thick, raised and lumpy and remain within the boundaries of the wound.

Ice Pick Scar
Scar resulting from un-treated inflammatory acne. Narrow craters in the skin that appear like a needle or puncture which are deeper than they are wide. Often needs subcision, soft tissue filler and LASER resurfacing to help decrease appearance.

Inflammatory acne
Caused by immune reaction inside the follicle in response to infection of the oil gland with a virulent strain of *P. acnes* bacteria. Hence, sudden papules often occur.

Infundibulum
The hair follicle canal.

Insulin resistance
A condition in which the cells do not respond to the insulin to allow it to bind to the cell to help with the glucose delivery causing further stimulation of the pancreas to produce more insulin. When

this reaction occurs chronically, it results in the diagnosis of Type 2 diabetes.

Intercellular cement or intercellular matrix
The lipid complex between the cells in the epidermis.

Irritants
Substances that can cause localized inflammation. Irritant reactions are most often caused by a substance damaging the barrier function of the skin, and in skin care, they are mostly caused by peeling or keratolytic agents.

Isolaz
An acne treatment device designed to evacuate or suction out pores or extracted cysts and destroy the bacteria that causes acne. In this treatment, a gentle vacuum opens the extracted pustules while pulsed light kills the acne bacteria and decreases inflammation. Safe for all skin types, it treats inflammatory acne as part of the surgical treatment after extraction of pustules. Isolaz can also be used for the maintenance therapy.

Isotretinoin
Oral form of the retinoid, Vitamin A derivative, better known by its historic trade name, Accutane, is a chemotherapy agent approved for treatment of severe inflamed nodulocystic acne.

Jessner's Solution
A peeling formula mixture of salicylic, resorcinol and lactic acid developed by dermatologist Dr. Max Jessner. Jessner's peels are probably the most dramatic peels used to reduce dark pigmentation.

Keloids
Hard, raised, dense scars due to a genetic disorder in which the skin makes excessive collagen as a reaction to skin injury, forming nodules which often lobulated like grapes and extend beyond the boundaries of the wound in contrast to hypertrophic scars which are a normal skin reaction to injury and remain confined to the boundaries of the wound.

Keratin
A protein which helps make skin resilient and helps prevent epidermal dehydration by sealing the skin's moisture.

Keratinocytes
Skin cells in the epidermis that produce and are filled with keratin.

Keratohyalin
A substance within epidermal cells which produces keratin.

Keratolytic
Class of ingredients that break up cell buildup helping loosen and remove blockages that occur in the follicles because of retention hyperkeratosis. Keratolytic products are used to break loose existing impactions, as well as preventing further accumulation of cell buildup in the follicle and on the skin surface.

KTP LASER
KTP stands for Potassium Titanyl-Phosphate. The KTP laser is used to treat blood vessels on the face, redness from rosacea and post-inflammatory erythema.

Lamellar granules
Specialized structures within the granular layer that produce lipids which eventually fill the gaps between the cells in the epidermis and regulate the sloughing rate of the corneum both on the surface and within the follicle.

Lamellated corpuscles
Pressure sensitive nerves in the skin.

Langerhans cell
A type of immune cell which roams through the mid-epidermis and dermis. The Langerhans cell's function is to detect and identify foreign bodies in the skin and to signal biochemical reactions that cause the skin and the body's systems to react to these foreign bodies.

LED
Treatments that expose the skin to light emitting diodes used as an

effective adjunctive treatment which kills bacteria inside follicles, decreasing inflammation and reduces swelling in the follicles.

Lesion counts
a dermatological technique of counting actual lesions on patients' faces to track progress in treating acne conditions.

Levulan
The brand of a topical medication known as 5-aminolevulinic acid. This photosensitizing agent is applied to the skin in photodynamic therapy. This acid is pain free on application and causes the skin to become receptive to an activating light source.

Linoleic acid
Linoleic acid is a polyunsaturated omega-6 fatty acid and is one of two essential fatty acids for humans, who must obtain it through their diet. It is used in the biosynthesis of cell membranes and prostaglandins, which help regulate inflammation.

Lipase
An enzyme which breaks fats into smaller components.

Lipophilic
Literally means "fat-loving", used to describe ingredients that are attracted to fats.

Lobes
Sections of a sebaceous gland in the skin that contain sebocytes, or oil-producing glands.

Macules
Flat discolored marks left from former acne lesions.

Malpighian cells
Cells within the stratum spinosum.

Meibomian glands
A type of sebaceous gland located in the upper and lower eyelids. They are distinguished by grape-like clusters of acini on the mucocutaneous lid junction, and empty their lipid content (sebum) to coat

the ocular surface via holocrine breakdown. Infection of these glands can present as inflamed cystic acne lesions.

Mechanical exfoliation
Physically removes dead cell buildup from the skin surface by literally "sloughing" them off the skin surface.

Meissner's corpuscles
Nerves that sense deep touch.

Melanocytes
Pigment-producing cells, located in the papillary dermis as well as the basal layer.

Melanosomes
Pigment granules produced by the melanocytes.

Melasma
Also known as Cholasma and "the mask of pregnancy", is hyperpigmentation caused by hormonal imbalances stimulating over-production of facial melanin.

Menopause
A time in a woman's life when menstration stops permanently.

Menstruation
Shedding the of uterine wall in the absence of pregnancy at the end of female's monthly menstrual cycle.

Microbiome
Normal variety of naturally-occurring bacteria found within an area of the body which protect the skin.

Microcomedone
A microscopic "clumping" of corneocytes in the lower sebaceous follicle, forming a plug-like structure that is the beginning of comedonal acne

Microdermabrasion
An office-based procedure that uses gentle mechanical abrasion combined with suction to remove the outermost layer of dead skin.

Often used to improve mild skin texture irregularity due to wrinkles or atrophic acne scars.

Mineralocorticoids
Steroids which help to regulate mineral content in the blood.

Multi-factorial
Describes a process that involves many different factors in order for the process to take place.

Nodule
A very deep lesion, similar to a papule, only much deeper in the dermis, and can even reach the subcutaneous layer of skin. Nodules can form when the rupture in the follicle wall is very deep in the structure.

Noncomedogenic
Refers to products and ingredients that have low or no potential to cause follicular blockage leading to whitehead and blackhead formation.

Non-essential amino acids
Amino acids that can be manufactured by the body.

Non-inflammatory acne lesions
Open and closed comedones which are not inflamed or red.

Occupational acne
Acne that is associated with exposure to certain acnegenic substances in the work place.

Ocular rosacea
Presents as redness and capillary dilation in the eyes and eyelid skin. Persons with ocular rosacea have frequent problems with styes (hordeolums), lumpy cysts in the lids known as chalazia, red eyes, thickened eyelids, and redness around the eyes. Persons with ocular rosacea often also have another subtype of rosacea.

Oil absorbers
Products that contain special ingredients such as silica and nylon that help to absorb excess oil.

GLOSSARY OF TERMS & DEFINITIONS

Omega-3 fatty acids and omega-6 fatty acids
Known as the essential fatty acids meaning they must be ingested because they cannot be produced by the body Itself.

Open comedones
Also known as blackheads, these are dilated follicles filled with a solidified plug of dead cells and sebum. The black plug is due to presence of oxidized melanin.

Ovaries
The main sex organ in females.

Over-the-counter (OTC) drugs
Chemicals and Drugs deemed safe enough for consumer use without physician's supervision and they contain non-prescription drug ingredients approved by the FDA.

Ozone
Heavy form of oxygen, O_3. Ozone Is also known for its antimicrobial properties.

Pancreas
Visceral organ that produces gastric enzymes to break down food, as well as insulin to regulate blood sugar.

Papilla
A large structure at the bottom of the hair follicle where hair growth originates.

Papillae
Fingerlike projections at the top of the papillary dermis.

Papillary dermis
Connects the dermis and the epidermis and is located between the reticular dermis, and the epidermis.

Papule
A round elevation of skin less than 1 cm, often with no visible fluid or pus. Can be brown, purple, pink or red in color.

Papulopustular rosacea
Subtype of Rosacea that most resembles acne. It is characterized by large red papules and pustules that are primarily in the nose and upper cheek areas.

Perimenopause
Describes the period of time around menopause, and can be as many as 10 years in duration where the menstrual cycle becomes extremely irregular due to significant hormonal shifts. This period of time is also when some adult women can experience exacerbation of their inflamed cystic acne or new comedonal eruptions.

Perioral dermatitis
Acne-like condition that effects women between the ages of 20 and 50. It is believed to be hormonally related and presents as clusters of acneiform (acne-like) red papules around the mouth. Occurs primarily in women during childbearing years. It effects maily the lower face and sometimes the nose.

Photodynamic Therapy (PDT)
A non-invasive therapy that utilizes blue light treatment in combination with the application of the phosensitizing agent, typically aminolevulinic acid (brand name Levulan). PDT has also been shown to be a safe and effective treatment for acne by shrinking oil glands and killing the acne bacteria.

Photoaging
Significant sun damage that destroys dermal collagen and results in premature aging of the face.

Phymatous rosacea
Affects primarily the nose with redness and in long-term and severe cases, growth and thickening of the nasal cartilage resulting in enlargement of nose itself, a condition known as rhirophyma.

Pituitary gland
Located in the center of the head, is the "master gland" and secretes hormones that signal other endocrine glands to make other hormones.

Plethoric
redness in the face seen in pregnancy due to increased blood flow and vascular congestion.

Polycystic Ovarian Syndrome (PCOS)
Group of conditions caused by severe hormonal imbalances including high levels of androgens resulting in numerous symptoms and conditions, including severe and chronic acne.

Post Inflammatory Hyperpigmentation (PIH)
Darkening of the skin occurring after inflammation or damage to the skin, such as an acne cyst or trauma or manipulation to the skin. It can last weeks to months and fades slowly, and can be treated by peels, creams or LASER therapy. This condition is more common in darker skin patients.

Post-inflammatory Erythema
Redness occurring on the skin at the site of trauma or manipulation. Often occurs after an acne cyst or pimple. Can occur after manual manipulation of the skin. Generally, fades over time, but can be decreased by LASER therapy. This condition is more common in lighter skin patients.

Polysaccharides
Carbohydrates made of chains of sugar unit molecules.

Pomade acne
A specific type of acne characterized by small bumps around the hairline and forehead, thought to be caused by use of greasy or waxy hair styling gels.

Pore
Refers to the appearance of the follicle opening when looking at the surface of the skin (plural: ostia).

Post-inflammatory hyperpigmentation (PIH)
Hyperpigmentation that occurs after an irritation or injury to the skin which cause inflammation.

Progesterone
Another prominent female hormone produced by ovaries which can be converted to testosterone.

Propionibacterium acnes (*P. acnes*)
The primary bacteria in the follicles which is part of the skin's microbiome and forms the skin's protective acid mantle. A virulent and opportunistic strain is thought to be responsible for pustular acne formation due to infection of the oil glands.

Proteins
Chains of molecules of amino acids, which are used by every cell of the body to carry out various functions as required by the cells and the body.

Proteolytic enzymes
Proteins that dissolve proteins. In skin care, they are used in surface exfoliation products. Three primary types of enzymes are used in epidermal exfoliation are papain derived from the papaya plant. bromelain extracted from pineapple, and pancreatin is derived from beef or pork pancreas as a side product of meat processing.

Puberty
The time of life when a child's body begins sexual maturity and significant hormonal changes.

Pus
A fluid comprised of millions of white blood cells mixed with follicular debris and inflammatory soup.

Pustule
An inflamed, round, elevated bump in the skin containing pus similar to an abscess, which can be opened or extracted to drain and disinfect.

Receptors
Specialized sites on the cell membrane or within the nuclear DNA of a cell that accept signals to make hormones.

Red Light Therapy
A light treatment within the 500nm visible light range, used for

reducing inflammation. Red light can help speed up healing time after procedures and can decrease post-inflammatory erythema associated with acne.

Resorcinol
A chemical that has antiseptic and keratolytic properties, and can increase penetration of the skin for other agents such as chemical peels as in Jessner peel. It is also combined with sulfur in some topical acne-treatment products.

Rete pegs
The top sides of the papillae.

Retention hyperkeratosis
An inherited genetic condition in which dead corneocytes fall to shed normally from the skin, resulting in follicular plugging that can lead to acne lesions.

Reticular dermis
Comprises the largest part of the dermis, containing collagen, blood vessels, and nerve endings. It sits just above the subcutaneous layer.

Retinoids
Derivatives of vitamin A. They are used in topical preparations in both esthetics and dermatology.

Rolling Scars
Depressed, atrophic acne scars on the skin that have a wavy texture.

Rosacea
A common, non-contagious genetic vascular condition that results in diffuse redness, large acne-like pustules and papules, facial swelling, dilated and distended capillaries, and in chronic cases, skin thickening. There are 4 subtypes of rosacea.

Salicylates
A class of naturally-occurring compounds that include salicylic acid, used as a keratolytic and anti-inflammatory in acne products

Salicylic acid
FDA-approved OTC acne-active ingredient, also referred to as beta-hydroxy acid. It is derived from willow tree and works by loosening dead cell buildup in the follicle and reducing inflammation.

Sebaceous follicles
The largest in diameter and deepest of all three types of follicles and have much larger sebaceous glands. Acne develops in sebaceous follicles.

Sebaceous gland
Small gland in the skin attached to follicles that secretes a yellow oil matter called sebum, which lubricate the hair follicles, hydrates (seals) and makes the skin waterproof. Often collects bacteria, is the main substrate for follicular bacteria and is the site of pustule formation when the oil glands are infected with a virulent strain of *P. acnes* bacteria.

Sebocytes
Cells which secrete sebum.

Seborrhea
Overabundance of sebaceous secretions resulting in extremely oily skin.

Seborrheic dermatitis
A condition of the skin that presents as red, flaking or scaly dry-looking skin is actually an inflammation of the sebaceous glands and is only found in oily areas. It is commonly seen in the eyebrows, hairline, scalp, ears, forehead, and the sides and corners of the nose.

Sebum
A fatty complex that flows through the follicles and lubricates the surface of the skin.

Silica and nylon
Ingredients used in products to help control excess surface skin oiliness.

Simple sugars
Present in table sugar (also known as sucrose), fruit sugars (fructose), and milk sugars (lactose).

Spironolactone
A prescription drug, also known as Aldactone, which is sometimes used to treat hormonally related acne. It is used an anti-androgen because it blocks the testosterone receptor cells on the sebocytes / oil-producing cells to prevent stimulation by dihydrotestosterone to produce oil.

Squalene
A colorless poly-unsaturated hydrocarbon liquid that's found naturally in many animals and plants, including human sebum. Essentially, it's one of the many natural lipids the body produces to lubricate and protect the skin. It is a highly-effective emollient and natural antioxidant.

Squalene oxidation
Oxidation of squalene in human sebum by bacteria or environmental pollutants is theorized as the trigger for eruption of inflamed sebaceous glands which present as acne cysts and pustules in humans.

Starches
Also called complex carbohydrates, are present in many vegetables including potatoes and rice.

Steroids
Well-known type of hormones named for their chemical Structure which are used for communication within the organs and cells of the body.

Strata
Sub-layers of the epidermis.

Stratum corneum
The outermost layer of the epidermis.

Stratum granulosum
Also known as the granular layer, located above the stratum spinosum.

Stratum lucidum
An extremely thin epidermal layer on the hands and feet between the granular layer and the corneum.

Stratum spinosum
Located just above the basal layer sometimes called the spiny layer.

Subcutaneous layer
Also known as the subcutis, makes up the very bottom layer of the skin and is basically a layer of fat that provides cushioning between the upper layers of skin and the muscle layer that lies below.

Sudoriferous glands
Glands in dermal layer of the skin that secrete sweat to help regulate body temperature.

Sulfur
Works as a keratolytic and peeling agent, helping to clear follicles and dry up individual acne blemishes. Sulfur also is believed to somehow block the breakdown of sebum into free fatty-acids, which are known to cause inflammation. Therefore, sulfur is a good addition when redness is an issue.

Surfactants
Cleansing agent ingredients that help to reduce the surface tension, allowing easy removal of oils, dirt, and other debris on the skin surface. Surfactants are sometimes called detergents. Overuse of surfactants such as soaps to wash the skin, strips the skin of protective oil and forces the skin to make more oil which can exacerbate acne.

Target cells
Cells that contain specific receptors for a specific hormone.

Tazarotene
A synthetic retinoid topical prescription drug used as a keratolytic. Also used to treat psoriasis and photoaging.

Telangiectasias
Dilated capillaries, spider veins, often seen in Rosacea.

Terminal follicles
The deepest follicles that contain beardtype hairs.

Testes
The main sex hormone and sperm producing organ in males.

Thyroid
Gland which secretes hormones to regulates growth and metabolism.

Transepidermal water loss (TEWL)
Evaporation of water or moisture from the epidermis.

Tretinoin
Sometimes called retinoic acid, but better known as the trademarked name Retin-A, is a vitamin A derived acid. It is used in skin products to increase skin cell turnover.

Triggers
Refer to aggravating and environmental factors that cause flares of rosacea

Trophic hormones
Hormones that signal other endocrine glands to make other hormones.

Tumors
Thick masses of tissue

Vascular macules
Red marks left on the skin after the acne lesions have resolved. This redness is caused by still-dilated blood vessels.

Vegans
Diet consisting of strictly plant products with no animal or dairy products.

Vellus follicles
The shortest follicles that produce tiny "peach fuzz" hairs.

Whitehead
Closed comedone containing sebum, keratin, dead cells and floral bacteria. No clinical inflammation is present. Pore remains white or yellow as it is covered by a layer of skin and not exposed to air.

CPSIA information can be obtained
at www.ICGtesting.com
Printed in the USA
FSHW021200270320
68540FS